The Back Story *on* Spine Care

A SURGEON'S INSIGHTS
ON RELIEVING PAIN AND
ADVOCATING FOR THE
RIGHT TREATMENT TO
GET YOUR LIFE BACK

Dr. Drew Bednar

DISCLAIMER

All cases described in this book are composites of true events. Some names and identifying details have also been changed to protect patients' right to confidentiality and privacy. Some cases are based on my own practice, and some come from concerned colleagues around the world. None of these cases is overly exceptional. Spine surgeons encounter the issues you'll read about here regularly. No client found in this book corresponds to any actual person, living or dead.

Published by ECW Press
665 Gerrard Street East
Toronto, Ontario, Canada M4M 1Y2
416-694-3348 / info@ecwpress.com

Cover design: Jessica Albert

LIBRARY AND ARCHIVES CANADA CATALOGUING IN PUBLICATION

Title: The back story on spine care : a surgeon's insights on relieving pain and advocating for the right treatment to get your life back / Dr. Drew A. Bednar.

Names: Bednar, Drew A., author.

Description: Includes index.

Identifiers: Canadiana (print) 20230236960 | Canadiana (ebook) 20230236995

ISBN 978-1-77041-728-1 (softcover)
ISBN 978-1-77852-206-2 (ePub)
ISBN 978-1-77852-208-6 (Kindle)
ISBN 978-1-77852-207-9 (PDF)

Subjects: LCSH: Backache—Treatment—Case studies. | LCSH: Backache—Patients—Rehabilitation—Case studies. | LCSH: Spine—Surgery—Case studies. | LCGFT: Case studies.

Classification: LCC RD771.B217 B43 2023 | DDC 617.5/64—dc23

This book is funded in part by the Government of Canada. *Ce livre est financé en partie par le gouvernement du Canada.* We also acknowledge the support of the Government of Ontario through the Ontario Book Publishing Tax Credit, and through Ontario Creates.

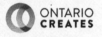
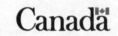

PRINTED AND BOUND IN CANADA   PRINTING: MARQUIS   5   4   3   2   1

Contents

PART 2   WHEN SURGEONS FAIL THEIR PATIENTS

PART 3   SPINE CARE SOLUTIONS

Preface

The Shocker — My First Encounter with the Realities of Modern Spine Care

I t was 1988 and I was a board-certified orthopedic spine surgeon practicing in a university teaching hospital. Finally! It had taken a long time to get here: college, a pre-med year, four years in med school, a year of surgical internship, four more training in orthopedics and then a year of fellowship specializing in spine care. Didn't sleep much or know my wife very well and could only recognize the twins on a good day but *damn!* I knew the spine. *I was ready!*

I had no idea what was coming.

∫

I'd just dozed off after an adrenaline-filled day of operating, seeing patients and triaging surgery, all while teaching medical students, residents and fellows. Got home, looked in on my sleeping kids, kissed my wife and crashed. Didn't even think about eating a late dinner before heading for my pillow.

The page came at 11:30 p.m. The chief of neurosurgery needed *my help* with a case. The *chief* no less! A teenager had fallen out of a tree and broken her back. The injury was the dreaded *burst* fracture where the vertebrae, the spine bones, are compressed so violently they literally explode. The patient was partially paralyzed by bone fragments crushing her spinal cord. The chief was going to try to reverse the paralysis by surgically removing all those bone fragments, doing what's called a *posterolateral decompression*, but he needed my specialized expertise to stabilize the fracture with the then-new screw-and-rod implants that he didn't know how to use. *Did he want me right away?* No, he wanted to start the surgery and do his part but would call for me when he was finishing. Great, I had a few hours to sleep.

Sleep my eye. I was way too excited. But I tried. When the pager went off again at 4:00 a.m., I jumped out of bed, dressed and took off like a shot for the hospital. I think I kissed my wife but might not have. The roads were empty and even the coffee shop in the hospital lobby was closed.

At the OR, I was surprised to find no sign of the chief; he'd done his thing and gone. There were no X-rays up. Likely he'd left them in the ER. The patient was asleep, the wound open but covered with sterile towels. I quickly looked over the surgical instrument trays and the right equipment was all there. I put on my special magnifying operating glasses and scrubbed in while asking for a second dose of antibiotics to be given, since the patient had already been open for four hours.

I lifted off the sterile towels and gently suctioned away the clotted blood to expose the surgical field. Eventually, I could clearly see what was left of the surrounding bony anatomy and the spinal cord exposed within it. My vision blurred, bile rose in my throat and I felt my heart skipping beats in my chest.

During surgery we don't commonly see the actual spinal cord or nerves themselves; we see the thin fibrous membrane that wraps around them to contain the spinal fluid. This is called the *dural membrane* or *dura*. It's an extension of the same membrane that wraps around the brain in the skull to protect it, and it ends just above your tailbone. Normally the dura is a small soft tubelike structure less than an inch in diameter.

This dura was flattened and stretched out over bone fragments underneath it, tight as a drum. So tight that it had no pulse. So tight that the spinal cord inside it likely had just about no blood flow. *After four hours of surgery? What the hell?* I started probing and dissecting right away; those fragments had to go. Why hadn't the chief pulled them out? Oddly, I found them to be smooth and rock solid — burst fracture fragments aren't usually like that. *This didn't make sense! What to do?*

I called for X-ray and the operating fluoroscope, and I saw that the spine was partially dislocated: one vertebral bone had been completely knocked out of joint and was in front of the other. Bone wasn't crushed, nothing had burst.

You don't fix a dislocation by decompressing it; you fix a dislocation by reducing it, by putting it back in joint. Imagine dislocating your ankle so violently that the blood vessels are kinked and cutting off the flow of blood to your foot. We don't save you from gangrene by operating for hours on the kinked blood vessels. We save your foot by quickly putting your ankle back in joint in the ER.

Why hadn't the chief done that in the OR with this spine?

I was a young idiot surgeon and I was thinking out loud way too much. The OR nurses and anesthetist started telling me how hard he'd struggled trying to do the decompression, even with the help of two assistants. He'd left unhappy and frustrated after doing his best.

In the surgical field, the bones are wet and slippery, and you can't hold them well with the hand, so we have to use surgical clamps of various sorts. With one clamp attached to the bones on either side of the fracture, I could easily pull the vertebrae apart a bit to "unlock" them, then manipulate them out of their dislocated position and back into place. When I released the clamps, everything stayed put.

The dura swelled up nice and round again and started to pulse. The fluoroscope confirmed that everything was well realigned. I probed and dissected, looking for any residual pressure on the neurological bits, and there wasn't any.

Still using the fluoroscope for guidance, as I had been trained to do, I set two great strong pedicle screws into each of the vertebrae on either side of the dislocation and secured them together with stainless-steel rods. After setting all the connectors tight, I harvested some bone graft from the patient's pelvis and did a fusion before closing the wound. In the recovery room, we found the patient's partial paralysis was actually a little bit better right away. Eventually, I learned years later, she did walk again.

Thanks to me. Not to that other jackass.

I was *pissed*! How could a chief of neurosurgery not recognize a dislocation? How could he be so incompetent? This was soooo wrong. I had to talk to the chief of surgery about it as soon as possible!

Expert though I was, I really was a young fool and heading for big professional trouble in the small community of the hospital. My anesthetist in the case, a very senior guy, saw it coming so he went out of his way to corner me in the changing room after the case and have a chat. It was suggested that I shut up and smarten up to keep my job. As it was, the halls would be awash with negative gossip for weeks with all the mouthing off I had already done about the Golden Boy's screwup. That anesthetist probably saved my career.

The sun was up when I left the OR. I went up to my office and did some paperwork, then spent some time looking at the sunny day outside the window and thinking about how nice it would be to enjoy days like that with my kids, but not today because I needed to sleep. I did need my job to support them. And so I decided to shut up.

I had been taught that the chief of any surgical service was always all-knowing and always right. Today I know that that old chief, a classically trained brain surgeon with only peripheral knowledge about the spine, was actually doing his best but working in ignorance. He lacked the knowledge to treat spine fractures properly. But his powerful position in hospital and university politics made it impossible for upstarts like me to confront that transparently. So

I stayed shut up and let him go on contributing to so much of the bad spine care that still goes on today.

But now it's time to talk.

WHY WRITE THIS BOOK?

Several times every year I am referred at least one patient who has either been deteriorating neurologically or is pretty much bedridden with an unstable mechanically impaired spine *despite having been under active medical care* for weeks or even months, often as a hospitalized inpatient. And it's an even bet I'll get another referral every other month about somebody who's had an operation and is worse off for it.

Pick a case. I alone have probably got a dozen just like it! Every missed case of myelopathy or spinal stenosis, the spine tumors and infections and unrecognized sciatica and even "emergencies" like cauda equina syndrome present to surgeons like me around the world pretty much the same way. These patients have often been under medical care for long periods of time, with their symptoms not recognized for what they are by physicians who have had little spine care training or by the paramedicals they seek out to ease their suffering, such as physiotherapists, chiropractors, kinesiologists and others.

For a long time, I thought all this was a function of Canada's unique health care systems, but it's not. Spine care colleagues across the world bemoan regularly encountering the same thing when we meet at conferences or share cases at rounds. Things like this should never happen in any modern health care system. I'd like to take a shot at changing some of that.

Spine surgery today should almost always be as awesome as one of my OR days in September 2022 was. Two people with badly pinched nerves in their backs from spinal stenosis (more later!) were so weak and rubbery and numb in their legs they could barely stand up and had been that way for some years, although neither had much back pain. He was 51, she was 78, and both were lurching through their lives as if they were a hundred. In four hours of surgery each, I unpinched seven nerves in him and eight in her. He went home smiling and standing tall that evening (OK, maybe he was a little nuts), and she was much stronger and discharged the next morning as scheduled.

I'm hoping to help improve spine care by telling some of those difficult patient stories from everyday real-world spine care practice. Some of the cases are my own, but many aren't and come from friends and colleagues around the world. This is all stuff that comes into a spine surgeon's office or clinic every day, including common degenerative disease, metastatic tumors and infections. I'm not worried that patient X, Y or Z might feel identified, because the stories are so often the same, year after year after year.

I've given my patients fairly Anglo-Saxon names because I'm lazy, but Tom and Mary could just as easily be, and often are, Luigi or Hong Su or Konyushi or Mohammed or Vladimir or Hans or you pick it. These cases don't get much press and are never presented from the podium at the scientific meetings I attend, but they're always shared afterwards when we spine care surgeons gather at dinner, around the table at coffee break or in the hotel bar.

The case studies at the heart of the book are presented in Parts 1 and 2, coming from primary care doctors or surgeons respectively. If the stories of these patients help just one reader, be they patient or physician or Joe Public, to identify one future case and help that person avoid a spine care catastrophe — what I call a *spine crime* — it'll all be worth it.

Each of the first two parts concludes with a summary of the most common spine crimes and suggestions that could minimize them considerably. Part 3 goes on to offer further recommendations for how to improve the practice of spine care through better education, and it offers patients themselves tips on prevention — a little self-care for the spine. Some of the professional measures I propose may be controversial — doctors, and their affiliate societies and professional organizations, really don't like to be told what they should do — but they go to resolving the very real, debilitating problem of spine crimes. These are the medical education "cures" that I can only daydream about right now. I wish!

In closing, there is an appendix, The Influencers, which talks about some of the medical giants and mentors I have been lucky enough to study under and who have been instrumental in shaping my thinking not only about spine care but also patient care in the broader sense. There is also a lengthy section of Selected References at the back of the book, organized by chapter. Although this isn't a medical textbook, and I don't want it to be, the technical material I cover does have to be substantiated. For the curious patient or general reader, I have also provided brief annotations in plain English to give you some idea of what these books and articles cover. There's a world of information on spine care out there if you wish to explore the literature further.

WHO AM I ANYWAY?

The alpha spine surgeon today uses an intraoperative CT scanner linked to a virtual 3-D imaging and navigation platform and a surgical robot to reconstruct your spine with custom implants made on a 3-D printer, all using a minimally invasive technique. They do this with active neurological monitoring technology, checking your neurological function continuously to avoid paralysis.

That's not me.

As a spine fellow in specialty training in 1987, I learned to do just two things really well. One was to accurately insert screws to the pedicles of your spine without either drilling out the adjacent nerve roots or poking the screws into the aorta, the great blood vessel that lies right up against the front of the spine. The other was to do that percutaneously, through a quarter-inch cut in the skin and with X-ray assistance. Almost nobody in the world could do that back then.

That's not me today either.

My professional title is Clinical Professor of Orthopedic Surgery at McMaster University in Hamilton, Ontario, Canada.

I was born and raised in Montreal and don't come from a medical family background at all. My dad was a telephone repairman for Bell Canada, and my mom was a school secretary. I went to a public high school and somehow managed to be The Smart Kid. After the next two years in Quebec's required public college program (they call it CEGEP), where I took the science stream, I was considering a career as a chemist when I realized I might be stuck in a lab looking at test tubes all day and never talk to another person. So, I put science and people together and applied to medicine. In the 1970s life was that simple.

After basic medical (MDCM, 1982) and orthopedic specialty (FRCSC, 1987) training at McGill University, I completed a year (1987–88) of specialized Spine Surgery Fellowship training at the University of Toronto under Drs. John Kostuik (who later moved on to be chief of spine at Johns Hopkins and from there founded a successful multinational spine implants company called K2 Medical) and Stephen Esses (who went on to be chairman of orthopedic surgery at Baylor in Houston). I'm board-certified in both Canada and the USA. The States makes you recertify every 10 years so I've actually done five board exams (six, if you count the one that my home province of Quebec requires for practice there).

All my practice has been in Hamilton, where I've now worked clinically and academically since 1988. In that time I've accumulated over 60 peer-reviewed scientific publications and presented almost 200 scientific lectures and exhibits at spine care conferences around the world. I also act as a reviewer of scientific articles being considered for publication for several of the lead academic journals in my field today. God only knows how many lectures I have listened in on, articles read and upgrade courses taken.

Five things have driven me to keep studying and learning in my field for all those years. Two were my key teachers, Drs. Joseph Miller and John Kostuik (you can read more about the people who influenced my career heavily in the appendix). A third was Dr. Hamilton Hall who invited me to join the prestigious International Society for the Study of the Lumbar Spine five years into my practice. It is a great honor to be a member of one of the lead spine research societies in the world and what an education it has been, across all the spine disciplines — not just surgery! A fourth is the unmitigated carnage too often practiced on the public by surgeons who spend a year learning nothing more than how to do procedures (that's called *fellowship*) and then stop learning as soon as they have that practice license to print money. Last is what I see as the great need for spine care issues to be presented in simple and understandable terms — only then can we communicate the issue well to our patients and our peers.

I am an active member of numerous major academic orthopedic and spine societies including the Canadian Orthopedic Association, the American Academy of Orthopedic Surgery, the Canadian Spine Society, the North American Spine Society, the International Society for the Study of the Lumbar Spine, the AO Spine group and the International Society for the Advancement of Spine Surgery, among others. In all this, my focus and interest remain not in academia or the lucrative business of technology development but in the optimally effective and seamless delivery of care — surgical or otherwise — to the spine care patient.

Spine surgery is very high-tech today; computers are everywhere and both artificial intelligence and virtual reality are on their way into the operating room. All this tech is very cool, but it can attract surgeons away from the basics. Too many academic spine surgeons hook up to industry and technology, then seem to have their focus sidetracked by the financial benefits and obligations that come with that.

Practicing in Canada at a university not known for a lead role in spine care has protected me from some of those compromising opportunities. I'm basically just a guy interested in accurate diagnosis and efficient, effective spine care. I have to be in Canada's eroded socialized health care system! We have no beds for you to stay in and no beds to admit complications to, very little OR time for your treatment, be it complicated or not, so there's been a huge practical advantage to my practice in putting in the time and effort to understand how to do what I do accurately and well. Again, I'd like to share some of that here.

Over many years of study and practice, I have assembled enough knowledge to figure out and communicate to my patients in an understandable and accessible way a scientifically based "model" or understanding of the spine: how it works, what can go wrong with it and what's involved in clinical spine surgery. My hope is that by sharing my knowledge and experience in this book with a broader audience of both general and medical readers, I can demonstrate how much better my field of adult spine care and surgery could and should be, and how it could be driven to evolve in that direction.

Introduction

Back Basics — A Brief History of Modern Surgical Spine Care

The opening line of Charles Dickens's classic book *A Tale of Two Cities* reads, "It was the best of times, it was the worst of times." Certainly, the last three decades in spine care *have* been both the best and worst of times. Excellence in surgical and nonsurgical spine care has very much been a moving target — but the good news is that at the leading edge of surgical spine care knowledge, we are closer to the bullseye than we have ever been. The journey was never finished in Dickens's story, and this tale may never be done either.

When I started my training in spine care in the late 1980s, what we could do was very limited, primitive and uncertain in outcome even after almost a century of practice. Understanding the history of how that could be, and what's been learned since, has helped me figure it all out a great deal.

Surgical spine care had arguably gone mainstream in 1911 with two almost back-to-back articles published out of Boston by Drs. Albee and Hibbs, both of which told the world that spine fusion surgery could relieve back pain. Wow! Up till then, neurosurgeons might fish out the occasional spine tumor, and most orthopedic surgeons did almost nothing in the spine. The "scientific" journals of the day actually argued as to whether *any* bone surgery was *ever* warranted! Orthopods like me were pretty much bonesetters of fractures or amputators of limbs, but all of a sudden these two authors gave bone surgeons an elective surgical care option for the patient with a painful joint or limb — we could do a fusion! Fusion surgery outside the spine took off like a rocket and is still done commonly throughout the skeleton to good effect today, though we've since developed motion-preserving replacements for most of the body's joints.

Spines are a bit more complicated than arms and legs, however, and it turns out that fusions for simple back pain don't work too well. Albee and Hibbs had reported the results of spine fusion on patients with scoliosis or tuberculosis, both conditions that can erode the strong support structure of the spine to the point of collapse. It was unrecognized at the time, but they were in effect operating on that instability (fusion brings strength and stability to the spine), which brought relief to people with certain conditions. Unfortunately, patients with "just" backache and some worn-out discs on an X-ray — that is, without neurological compressions, an unstable structure or a deformity — are today described as having *back-dominant pain* and many surgeons feel (and, sadly, teach!) that these people can't be helped.

So, with most patients who underwent fusion operations continuing to suffer from back pain, our professional enthusiasm tanked within a decade and spine surgery waffled for almost a quarter century. Then, in 1934, Drs. Mixter and Barr, one a pathologist and one a neurosurgeon and both again out of Boston, published their landmark article in the *New England Journal of Medicine*, explaining that the pain of sciatica can be caused by disc hernia pinching nerve roots.

Overnight the spine surgical world changed. Spine surgery went from being the orthopedic bone surgeon's domain, with uncertain outcomes, to a soft-tissue neurosurgical thing where decompressing the neurological elements of the spine was everything. The

"Dynasty of the Disc" was founded, and bone surgery of the spine was sidelined. Today there are still surgeons who don't believe that anything other than disc hernia or neurological compression can be important in the spine. I've worked with some and conferenced with too many. There remains a terrible competitive schism between *neurospine* and *orthospine* practice, which does no good for anybody.

When a Dutch neurosurgeon named Henk Verbiest presented to the world at a 1949 surgical conference in Paris the concept that nerves could be compressed by bony narrowing of the main nerve channel (what's called today *central* spinal stenosis), the surgical world of the time refused to believe it because the Dynasty of the Disc was already so entrenched as dogma. It was fully five years before he got an article published, and that was in a journal outside his specialty — the *Journal of Bone and Joint Surgery*!

Through the 1970s European surgeons (particularly in Italy) went on to develop the associated concept of bony narrowing in the lateral nerve channels (lateral spinal stenosis) and how to treat it.

That's where adult surgical spine care for degenerative disease was when I started my training. My teachers in my junior years might remove the odd disc bulge, enlarge the spinal canal with a laminectomy operation that removes part of the posterior spine bone to open the neurological canal or trim a bone spur, but even that was rare. Heaven forbid a patient might need two spurs trimmed out; that needed a case conference and weeks of debate before a decision was made. Nobody was treated for arthritic or structural spine pain, and many were left in pain and disabled for want of care.

Bad outcomes gave spine surgery a terrible reputation and prompted decades of sad practice where too often even patients in dire need and terrible pain were warned against the surgical option. That still happens today! Instead of getting access to accurate diagnoses and surgical relief, these patients can be doomed to decades of "pain management," getting some (usually minor) respite with drugs, physical care (physiotherapy, chiropractic, osteopathy and the like), pain-relieving injections of various sorts and even psychotherapy. They suffer needlessly for not being referred to qualified specialist spine surgeons. Now don't get me wrong here, not for a second would I suggest surgery for your first twinge of backache. Only if symptoms have been present for at least many long months, maybe years, and are severe enough to cause major disability should spine surgery ever be considered. And again, don't get me wrong, all the nonsurgical stuff does work for pain in many cases and has a role — but too often it isn't effective. That's when surgery can help.

There have been two really revolutionary advances in adult surgical spine care through the years of my involvement in the field. OK, sure, there have been many more technologies developed through my time, but these are the biggies. The first came as I was finishing my training. Bolder surgeons had always done some occasional mechanical stabilizing work on patients with fractures and deformities using surgical wire or Harrington rods. Through the 1970s, it was recognized that those technologies didn't work very well for other kinds of spine trouble. French surgeons had been putting screws into their spine patients since the 1960s. In the late 1980s, these pedicle screws were imported to North America and we tried them out. I did some of the first pedicle screw cases at McGill University in my senior resident year, 1986–87. They were awesome!

Before the pedicle screw, we'd wrap some wires around a bone or balance a foot-long Harrington rod on your spine and pray they didn't break or dislocate from you coughing after surgery. A third of them did. All of a sudden we could set some great big screws in there (the things are commonly two inches long or more, and about a quarter inch in diameter), and we could *feel* the screws hold the bone tightly as we screwed them in. Wow! Spine fusion surgery with screw fixation exploded, and technology rapidly expanded to let us do it throughout the length of the spine. This was the best of times!

There were just a few teensy problems with all this. Early screw designs were frail, and they'd break or tear loose a lot. We had almost no idea of who best to do fusion for, how best to do it or what alignment might be good or bad for the patient. Like those backache patients who had simple bone graft fusions in the first few decades after Albee and Hibbs, a lot of people went through this fusion surgery and came out of it no better off — or worse! The problem was so big that it led to a massive class action lawsuit against this technology in 1994 that virtually shut down spine fusion surgery in the U.S. for two years. This was the worst of times.

The second earth-shattering advance in adult surgical spine care during my years of practice came in 2005 with the publication of a landmark article by Dr. Steven Glassman reporting on adult deformity surgery. Adult deformity is the ultimate last stage of disc degeneration; the spine becomes so worn out it literally collapses on itself. These are massive operations that can take all day and put patients in ICU for their aftercare — I might get one case done in the time my cardiac buddies do two or even three surgeries. Dr. Glassman's analysis proved that the single most important determinant of how these patients would do wasn't how badly off they were to start with or how thoroughly decompressed their nerves were by the surgery, but whether he got their alignment right or not.

This shouldn't have been rocket science. Fracture surgeons way back in the 1960s had recognized that setting your broken arms or legs straight before screwing them back together was a good thing (duh!), but until Glassman there was very little knowledge of, or research into, what an individual patient's ideal spinal alignment should be. Try standing bent forward or sideways a bit, pretty soon you're tiring and in pain from the strain on your muscles. Europeans had started thinking about this in the 1990s. After Glassman proved the importance of the concept, over a decade of research and technology advances was spawned. Today we can predict almost exactly what would best be done for the adult reconstructive spine patient.

How do we know that we've reached this point? Spine surgery has always had a bad reputation for bringing the patient back: "Don't have the operation, you'll need another and another and another . . ." Historically that's true, and the odds were defined as roughly 3 percent per year of life in another classic 1999 article by Dr. Alan Hilibrand. This has been repeatedly found in research from around the world since and was unchanged until we had enough follow-up on properly aligned fusion patients to prove otherwise. Dr. Rothenfluh in 2015 was among the first to show that we can cut the reoperation rate by almost 90 percent simply by "setting our patients straight." So, today should really be the best of times.

∫

There's a great joy in understanding where all these decades have brought my field, which comes to the surgeon meeting patients in need and in knowing that we can help so many. But there remains a terrible problem in modern spine care. This is not an issue of deficient knowledge or understanding or resources or cost containment. It's a lack of knowledge translation — spreading the news — in other words, taking all of this info and teaching it to the general physician population base who are best positioned to diagnose these problems early and to refer patients to qualified surgeons. My profession's failure to drive what we spine specialists know into the mainstream medical curriculum has led to a terrible knowledge gap that causes patients harm every day. So we may still be in the worst of times.

Too often we fail even to get surgical knowledge from our elite academic spine societies and journals to the common surgeon in practice. That chief of neurosurgery I came up against wasn't stupid or uncaring, but he was *ignorant* in the classical sense. He just didn't know the difference between a fracture and a dislocation. My issue is not with the highly competitive business, professional and academic marketplace competing on the question of how best to do things. The problem I see time after time is simple lack of knowledge and understanding of the fundamentals of spine care and patient assessment that identify who needs care and the basics of what needs to be done for them. That applies at the primary care level, to surgeons who operate on spines without specializing in the practice and, sadly, even to some spine surgeons.

The simple truth is medical learners today get very little spine care education, and so while expertise exists and can bring good outcomes to most spine care patients, most physicians simply have no knowledge of the options. Often they don't even know how to recognize these spine care problems when they encounter them, nor do they understand that surgery might help. I lectured once to a family doctors' group in a very upscale Toronto suburb on the subject of spinal stenosis, likely the most common indication for spine surgery today — and the group didn't know surgery was an option. I heard, "We send all that to the pain clinic."

Patients often don't get referred to us at all, and if they are, too often it's too late. As I worked on this book in March 2020, I had just recently operated on yet another 74-year-old woman whose legs had been getting weaker and weaker for over a decade while regular injections at the pain clinic dulled her pain and enriched her doctors but allowed her nerves to be more and more compressed to the point of withered muscles and a basic inability to stand and walk unaided. She's doing well now and is much stronger, but she'll never be normal; the scans and referral she needed were done way too late. In May 2020, I operated on four similar cases in just one week! As I rewrote again in September 2021, I'd just treated an even older lady who was in similar circumstance but worse off. She was so weak after years of being unable to stand and walk more than a few steps that she just withered away and died about six weeks after the surgery. I was too late to help her.

Today's medical learner gets all kinds of education about cardiac disease and cancer and HIV and a lot of other things, but by and large, the spine is not on the general medical radar very much at all. My own medical students at McMaster University are exposed to just 11 PowerPoint slides with the word *spine* on them and one backache case. The very small amount of research one can find on this unfortunate deficiency in medical education is all quite consistent.

Musculoskeletal problems generally, and especially spine care, are badly underrepresented in the medical curriculum.

I'm not asking that every doctor know what I do about the spine. Just a few simple things, the common early complaints. Sciatica, for example, is a symptom that can be caused by many things (more later), but most doctors never learn how it really presents. Patients commonly describe it as "my hip hurts." As a result, I've treated people who've actually had a hip replacement when their problem was really sciatica.

Even many surgeons are quite ignorant of the spine. In North America, every graduating orthopedic surgeon or neurosurgeon is expected to be qualified in only elementary surgical spine care for their board exams but is licensed such that they can legally do whatever spine surgery they want to. So, much if not most spine surgery today is done by people who spend most of their OR time doing other things. If your focus and study and lifelong learning efforts are not focused on the spine, it's really easy to become dated. Or to be swayed by a "scientific literature" that's too often not very scientific at all and is more about promoting fancy technologies and expensive treatments, and in which the underlying core principles of what we surgeons should be doing are often neglected.

And even spine surgeons can do better. We get a lot of training in how to "do things," but we learn little of the history and background of *why* we do what we do and spend very little time learning to interview and diagnose patients. We get virtually no training in biomechanics, kinetics, behavior, psychology and all the other things one needs for a comprehensive understanding of the modern spine care patient.

Professionally we know that's a problem, and efforts have been made to correct these deficits. In the U.S. there was an American Board of Spine Surgery that advocated for special training and certification for decades (it has folded into the North American Spine Society), and surgeons in several European countries have come together and developed the European Spine Care Curriculum (eccelearning.com), a wonderfully comprehensive program targeted at fully trained surgeons who want to optimize their spine knowledge and skills. But how many graduating surgeons, who have been living on slave wages for 10 or more years during their training, and have finally earned that medical license to print money and pay down their training debts, will take the time for that? Not a lot.

The best predictor of how the patient will do functionally and neurologically is always their condition when coming into the surgery. So, if I can return to quoting Mr. Dickens, while the expert knowledge we have in spine care today does make for "the best of times" — in that a truly expert surgeon will know what to do for the best outcome with a given patient — the fact that our physician colleagues and the paramedicals who might also refer cases to us don't have any of that knowledge still too often makes it "the worst of times" because the referral is so often too late.

Smart spine surgeons love to catch the neurological patient a bit numb and tingly, or the senior's spine when they're just starting to lose the ability to do what needs to be done in life — that's often a day surgery case whom we might never see again once the stitches are out. We hate to see a bedridden spastic patient or somebody who for years hasn't been able to stand or walk unassisted for 10 minutes. Those people often need complex long-term inpatient care and rehab, and while most improve a great deal, they almost never make a fully functional recovery. The worst is the poor patient who's had surgery delivered by somebody with not quite enough knowledge to treat the problem thoroughly and well and has just been made the worse for it.

The best evidence I can offer of this lack-of-knowledge problem is to reference a condition called *cervical myelopathy*, a common condition where age-related disc bulges and bone spurs in the neck crush the spinal cord to cause variable degrees of neurological loss and even paralysis. Research has suggested that one in four people over age 50 will show spinal cord compression in their neck MRIs, usually without symptoms but too often with. Some 50 years ago,

Dr. Harvey Nurick, in a 1972 article in the journal *Brain*, told the world that spine problems like this are a common cause of new-onset difficulty standing and walking in adults — but still today almost nobody knows that. It's not in the curriculum.

I see people with crippling spinal cord compressions in the neck all the time, who are worked up for fashionable rare neurologies like Guillain-Barré syndrome (GBS) or multiple sclerosis (MS), often getting worse for weeks and months before all that testing comes back negative and somebody says, "Gee, let's scan the neck." Guillain-Barré syndrome affects something like one in a million people, and cervical myelopathy affects hundreds! Too many of those people get worse while they're having all that misdirected workup.

If half of people over age 50 have some spinal cord compression, they obviously don't all need surgery, so there's an active field of research trying to identify who is at greatest risk for getting into trouble. There are two large recent population studies on this, one based in North America and the other in Eurasia. Between them they followed roughly a thousand asymptomatic people forward in time for a decade to see what would happen. The findings were that only 20 percent of patients got into trouble and so prophylactic (preventive) surgery is not indicated. But — and here I think is the most important take-home from this — the fine print in those articles reveals these patients from advanced countries around the world were, on average, neurologically symptomatic for between one and two years before even being *identified* as having a spinal cord compression. That's a problem. Nerve cells have been dying off, muscles getting weaker and coordination deteriorating for way too long before they find their way to a surgeon.

When it comes to spine care, the deficiency in modern medical education and practice is a great tragedy. But nobody's going to rewrite the world's medical school curriculum overnight, and if we did, it would still be a decade before informed physicians start graduating into practice in large enough numbers to help with all this. Concerned experts on the spine, specialist surgeons like myself, sometimes lecture and write articles targeting affiliate physician groups and other medical learners, but that's a very spotty and inadequate practice. With physician knowledge of just a few dozen key articles and some elementary spine biomechanics, the world of today's spine care patient would be a much better place. This info could be taught in just a few hours of lecture time! Is it important? You bet. People die, or worse. In Canada, one of the two people who went to our Supreme Court to get medically assisted suicide legalized had spinal stenosis — a very treatable and usually recoverable condition. That's sad.

People, physicians and patients both, should know the basics of spine care so patients can be referred to us in a timely way. That's why I wrote this book not just for a medical audience but for the general reader, so patients and their families might recognize trouble as it's happening and advocate for care. Remember all those people with asymptomatic spinal cord compression? The best thing to do for them is likely not just to remind their doctors that the spine could be a problem in the future, but for knowledgeable spine care practitioners to educate the patients themselves about the earliest symptoms of trouble so that they can present for care when it's due and well before it's too late.

Part 1

Primary Care Myths, Misdiagnoses and Missed Referrals

What family doctors, emergency physicians and other health care professionals need to know about spine care.

Chapter 1
John the Roofer

*A case of myelopathy. Spine care
isn't always about backache.*

John is usually a very nice guy. I meet a guy like him every other month or so. He can be young or old, thin or heavy, a working man or a pampered executive. But the front-end story is almost always something like this very real case of mine. In ignorance, doctors often make the same assumption that Joe Public commonly does in thinking that spine troubles must be horribly painful. Imagine all those raw nerve endings being compressed and irritated and inflamed . . .

But spinal cords don't have nerve endings in them, so they can often be badly damaged without much pain at all. Most doctors don't know that. So John's story and experience get repeated over and over again . . .

APRIL

"Murray! Look out!"

John had been roofing for almost 30 years, ever since he dropped out of school at 17. At first, this was easy work and great pay, 15 bucks an hour zipping up ladders with shingle bundles all day in the fresh air and the sunshine. Fifteen bucks! Overtime or not, back then it meant a nice apartment and cool wheels and life was good.

Thirty years later it wasn't so great anymore. John had a lot of aches and pains, and the pay hadn't gone up much. The worst thing was his numb hands that had been an issue for a year. It started with tingles at night that went away when he'd shake his hands back and forth, then there was tingling at work and then the numbness would wake him from sleep and now both his hands and arms felt numb all the time. When he dropped a shingle bundle again, halfway up the ladder, all he could do was shout a heads-up and hope that the boss wouldn't notice.

The bundle missed Murray below him and landed flat so it didn't break up. John zipped down past Murray and zoomed his bundle back up again with hands that felt dead. Shake shake shake, nothing. Maybe his wife, Chloe, was right and he should talk to the doctor about these hands.

JUNE

Getting a doctor's appointment in Canada is easy in a way — it's free — but boy do you wait for it. After dropping that bundle on his first job of the year in April, he got to the doctor in June. Got a whole four minutes' attention. His GP mumbled something about pinched nerves, didn't lay a hand on him and ordered a test called an EMG, electro-something-or-other, which was booked another month later. Wow! If the doctor was paid 10 dollars for seeing him, that's $150 per hour, and an eight-hour workday would mean $1,200. Nice for office work. John started to think that maybe he should have stayed in school too . . .

JULY

The test. In the hospital, he met a doctor in a nice white lab coat that said Neurology on it. They talked for five minutes; she examined him a bit and then stuck a bunch of electrodes on his arms and legs for a half hour. Afterwards, to her credit, the doctor actually had a talk with John, and he learned he had something called carpal tunnel syndrome, a pinched nerve in his wrist. Both wrists in fact. The doctor said that wearing a wrist splint might ease the pressure on his nerves. Most people wear it overnight when sleeping, but the more the better. *Why not?* The alternative was a surgical operation that would take him off work for at least six weeks. *Who can afford that in the busy summer roofing season?*

So John spent $40 he couldn't really afford and bought some splints. He wore them only at night so his boss wouldn't see he had a problem. They helped a bit with the nighttime symptoms and he slept better, but not much changed with the numb aching weakness affecting him from the shoulders down all day.

AUGUST

By now his hands were so numb he could barely hold onto the hammer. When he slowed down so he wouldn't drop it, the boss was on his back in a flash.

At break time he had 15 minutes to climb down the ladder, find some shade and chow down the lunch Chloe made him, thank God for that woman. Fifteen minutes later he was a bit rested and well fed, but his hands were still numb.

Here goes, back to work and back up to the roof, first rung, second . . . *Bam!* John is flat on his back at the bottom of the ladder, winded. His hands had become so numb he couldn't hold on.

He didn't pass out, but for a few seconds he felt numb and tingly all over and couldn't move. Then, as he sucked in that first big breath of air, he got some strength back in his arms and legs. But he could barely stand. Tingled like mad, arms and legs all sensitive to touch, and when he tried to walk over to the shingles pile to sit on it, his knees kept banging together, his legs kept crossing. Murray had to hold him up.

He still couldn't stand a half hour later. Boss was pissed and sent Murray off to do two men's work for one man's pay. After Chloe came to collect him, John wobbled into the truck and off to the ER where the doctor asked if he had pain, didn't examine anything and sent him for scans of his head and neck. Arthritis in the neck, normal head. Here's a pill for nerve pain, go see your family doctor if it's not better in a few days and maybe he'll send you for another scan or to see the neurologist again.

A week later John was still all tingly and wobbling. Mom's old walker helped him get around the house, but work wasn't going to happen any time soon. His family doctor said he needed an MRI scan of his neck and he might get it quickly because it's a compensation board case, maybe within a month or two. *Wow.* With bills to pay it was off to the comp board office, and he got a claim number. Murray said he'd witness the fall, and with that the comp lady said the first cheque might show in just a few weeks.

SEPTEMBER

The tingling was worse, but he was getting the hang of the walker thing. The MRI scan said his spinal cord might be pinched off by the arthritis, but they're not sure, so they want a repeat scan with some sort of intravenous dye before his GP might refer him to a surgeon for an operation that could kill or paralyze him. *Oh boy.* More waiting, and a blood test of his kidneys so the radiologist can dose the X-ray dye right.

Walker nothing, John's arms were now too weak to hold him up on it. He didn't have the strength to hold a cup of coffee! Chloe bought an old wheelchair on Kijiji. The second MRI scan was done in the first week of November, reported the next week and the report sent to his GP's office, but there was no appointment time until two weeks after that. So in early December, John learned he did have a pinched spinal cord and needed a surgeon. John had thought he was scared before; now he was terrified. *Surgery? What are my chances, Doc? Will I be paralyzed?*

Doc got all smirky and wouldn't say, just mumbled "I know a guy" and said he'd fax off a referral and call John with the appointment.

Two weeks later it's paperwork day at the family doctor's office and the referral fax finally gets sent. Now it's late December, offices and practices are closing for the holidays. Heck, the whole hospital closes to scheduled surgery for two weeks. So nothing happens until the New Year.

JANUARY

In the second week of the year, the doc's office called with a hospital clinic appointment on the next Friday. One o'clock, just after lunch. John and Chloe showed up to a crowd and waited it out till almost 3:00 p.m. before the surgeon saw them.

The surgeon's an odd duck, talked too much and wants to know about everything, even the carpal tunnel thing. He tried to examine John but it wasn't easy; because his arms and legs were so stiff, he couldn't move them around much. Then of all things the surgeon asked him to stand up and walk. *Why? The family doc never did that, neither did the neurologist.* John hauled himself erect, wobbled, leaned on the wall for balance and took a step forward, but the right leg he led with swung left and he just about fell over. The surgeon caught him and sat him back down.

The surgeon brought up the scan on the computer monitor and apologized for squinting at it for several minutes; there were a lot of pictures there. Wasted another five minutes bringing up the first scan as well, then squinted a bit more. He was able to look over the EMG test on the computer too. Left the exam room. Came back 10 minutes later with a long face and some forms. After explaining John's condition, he told him he'll never be normal again because things have gone on for so long and that he can't operate for at least two weeks because there are no beds and no OR time.

This was definitely not just carpal tunnel syndrome! What was really going on here?

THE ROOFER REVISITED

Transient numbness from neurological compression in a limb happens all the time and is generally benign. A common example is when your foot "falls asleep" while you're sitting with legs crossed. That happens from the weight of your leg compressing some sciatic nerve branches just above your ankle and cutting off their blood flow. Uncross your leg and you're fine in a minute or two, no long-term effects. There are several other points in the body where this happens similarly through positioning. The back of the upper arm (radial nerve) and the inner elbow (ulnar nerve) are others.

Numbness, rather than weakness or pain, is almost always the first symptom of nerve compression. Why? Anatomy — or more precisely, microanatomy. Under the microscope, we can see that a nerve is made up of thousands of longitudinal nerve fibers, rather like an old-fashioned telephone cable carrying hundreds of smaller wires. Some carry sensation (sensory), some control motion (motor) and a minority have other functions. The sensory fibers are much thicker than the motor fibers and the greater diameter makes them much more sensitive to external compression. You have to sit with your numb leg crossed for quite some time to challenge the smaller motor fibers — try it. I did, and it took me over 10 minutes to give myself a drop foot. But I was still without pain!

Pinched nerves don't hurt; inflamed nerves hurt. It likely takes several days of continuous compression for enough inflammation to build up in a nerve root to create pain.

There's a nerve in your palm called the median nerve, which crosses the wrist in a small anatomical space where it travels with several tendons of the big powerful forearm muscles that give your hands and wrists their strength. People who do regular heavy work with their hands have thicker stronger tendons in the wrist, just as they have bigger stronger muscles in the forearm, and so that space can get crowded and the median nerve, being softer than the tendons, is compressed. Voilà, carpal tunnel syndrome (or CTS in my heavily abbreviated medical world), a common workplace ailment causing numbness of the fingers.

The neurologist who first examined our roofer's numb hands didn't ask about the exact distribution of his numbness and did very little physical examination. Bad practice, but common in this day and age where basic anatomy is a smaller and smaller part of the medical school curriculum. She should have asked those questions because that distribution, the "where" of John's numbness, would have been a dead giveaway that this was much more than a simple carpal tunnel compression. The median nerve distributes to the palm side of the thumb, index, middle and half the ring finger as well as the back side of the corresponding fingertips. John's numbness involved not just the entirety of both hands but his arms up to the shoulders as well.

The pressure on the median nerve in the carpal tunnel varies with the position of the wrist. When you make a fist and grip tightly, your coiled fingertips and the base of your thumb tend to lie on a straight line paralleling the palm side of the forearm — that's the functional position of the hand. Pressure on the nerve is minimal here but goes up with either flexion or extension of the wrist from this point. That's why carpal tunnel syndrome commonly presents with nighttime symptoms: we often curl our wrists when we sleep, and they may stay that way through the night. When mine acts up, as it does once or twice a year, I'll wear a night splint that holds my wrist in the functional position overnight for a day or two. Works like a charm.

John the Roofer never complained of numbness in the classical carpal tunnel distribution. He had a touch of it, like I do, but had had that forever (like me) and could live with it, like I do. What he did complain of was new and increased numbness throughout the entire hand and even extending up the arms, classic spinal cord symptoms easily detected with just a few short words of conversation, old-fashioned "doctoring" which isn't very fashionable in the modern high-tech world.

The neurologist assumed (never assume!) common things are common and sought to confirm her CTS diagnosis with electrophysiological testing, whereby we send fine electrical signals into your nerves and see how they're carried along. EMG, or electromyography, tests the motor function in a nerve, and nerve conduction studies (NCS) are commonly used to test sensory function. These are arguably the gold standard tests for CTS, but they're not perfect and are commonly challenged by false positives, abnormal testing results where the patient might have few symptoms and no complaints.

Once the EMG test had "confirmed" John's CTS diagnosis, our neurologist ordered a wrist splint to be worn overnight. But not every wrist splint is a carpal tunnel splint. Too often I see people wearing Velcro splints that hold the hand straight on the forearm, forcing the wrist into a high-pressure flexed position and likely tending to *increase* CTS symptoms. Too many physicians just don't know any better for lack of anatomical knowledge and neurological education. A CTS splint has a stiff plastic or metal piece running on the palm side that should be bent to hold your wrist elevated into the functional position I described earlier (like a fist).

Why it *was* a spinal cord problem in the neck

John had more than just numbness; his hands and arms were weakening and he was dropping things even before he reached the point where he couldn't hang onto the ladder. But he *complained* of numbness. Doctors commonly assume the patient will pipe up and tell us accurately what all their symptoms are, but it's often not that simple — *we have to ask*. It's what "taking a medical history," as pioneered by the great Sir William Osler, is all about. This is another waning skill in today's high-tech age.

With prompting, the patient just about always tells me what their problem is even though they don't know or understand it. Simply asking the patient a few questions can reveal a great deal of information and help make an accurate diagnosis. Locating John's hand numbness would have quickly determined that CTS was not his issue.

To make matters worse, when John fell to the ground, his head snapped back and his neck likely wobbled a bit more than it safely could. The impact of motion-related bulging of the discs in his neck on his spinal cord increased his numbness to include the legs and increased his weakness to the point where for a few minutes he couldn't move anything at all. Technically, that's called a *transient quadriparesis*; in English, a temporary paralysis. Yes, that happens. In fact, it happens a lot; it's a big issue in American professional football, and I see it at least once or twice a year. It is commonly not recognized for what it is even when patients present with so much weakness they can't stand, walk or sometimes use their hands.

Temporary paralysis like John's happens from unguarded extremes of motion in the neck, such as might come on in a fall or from impact to the head. It won't happen in an anatomically normal neck. It happens only when the spinal canal is narrowed, either congenitally or more often from degenerative disc bulges and arthritis-related bone spurs. Normally the spinal cord is buried deep within the protective vertebrae, and the spinal fluid around it provides some "elbow room." This anatomy allows for transient disc and joint bulges, which are a normal part of physiologic motion, to safely impact on just the spinal fluid.

Some people are born with congenitally narrow or stenotic spinal canals where the spinal fluid bath is very thin or even absent. Massively strong heavy people can actually *develop* a stenosis from bony overgrowth or hypertrophy. Each vertebra is like a donut or a bagel surrounding the spinal cord, and a thicker donut has a smaller hole. That's the American football player: big heavy guy has big heavy bones. Transient quadriparesis is so common in that sport that spine care and sports medicine societies have put forward return-to-play guidelines, very similar to what is being developed for concussion today.

Most commonly, cervical stenosis is degenerative. Worn discs can bulge, and the bony facet joints in your spine commonly develop bone spurs, encroaching upon the spinal canal to narrow it. This occurs so often that classical MRI research found half of people over 50 years of age have a spinal cord compression — but only 10 percent of those present with a neurological problem.

Yes, a compressed spinal cord can be asymptomatic; spinal cords don't have nerve endings in them. They can't hurt! They can, in fact, tolerate a lot of pressure and deformation applied very slowly and gently, as through years of bone spur growth. What a spinal cord can't tolerate is sudden impact pressure. If an instrument slips in the OR and impacts the cord, that cord is toast. And when somebody with a stenotic neck has a fall or bonks their head, they can "quad out" quite commonly.

What was done right, or not?

To his great credit here, the family doctor knew that a very common cause of a new neurological deficit in an adult is spinal cord compression in the neck, cervical myelopathy, and appropriately ordered an MRI scan. What he didn't do was order an *urgent* MRI scan, or maybe even contact either the MRI radiologist or the on-call spine surgeon to potentially accelerate the care of his patient who had a suddenly increased neurological deficit. These are bad things, both the syndrome and the doctor's failure to "make the call" for urgency.

People with a critically compressed spinal cord often posture protectively. Involuntarily, they'll restrict motion (get stiff) or position their necks into flexion or whatever side-bend best opens their spinal canal to decompress the spinal cord a bit and relieve pain. These odd neck postures don't lend themselves to MRI scanning where we want the patient to lie down on their back in the machine remaining straight and still for several minutes. When the patient can't hold still, the radiologist gets blurred images that can be difficult to interpret, and in the absence of clinical info on point they might ask for a repeat scan or contrast enhancement (an IV dye injection) to improve the image quality. That was the case here, and it left our patient out there for several more months with a deteriorating compressed spinal cord. Who's to blame? Everybody, but more than anybody, the radiologist who was playing "I want a perfect scan" when he had a critical patient and more-than-adequate information on the first images to make the diagnosis.

So after another waiting list delay, the second scan was done and read as a severe spinal cord compression. You'd think the radiologist might pick up the phone and call somebody. He didn't, dropping the ball again, and so the report sat on a desk over the holidays and wasn't seen by the family doctor until the New Year.

Fax referrals may not always be a good thing; they can easily stack up in a spine surgeon's office in the dozens or even hundreds unless they all get looked over or triaged properly. (Yes, a lot of medical communication is still done by fax, even today!) In my opinion, a responsible surgeon should be reviewing those faxes at least once or twice a week. Too many can't or don't or won't: *We're busy, we're doing important research, we have meetings!* The actual patient care gets lost in the demands of managing a practice, academe and administration. Patient care is often seen as a minor thing within the modern hospital or university view — but if you'll chair all the meetings or get the Big Grant, you're *somebody*. I have plenty of spine colleagues who boast of one or two or even three years' worth of casework sitting in their offices. To me, that's simply irresponsible. Sadly, I've had to rescue more than one patient whose referral was buried in just such a pile of ignored paperwork when their neurological deficits went critical and the patient ended up in the ER.

What was the diagnosis? What was the surgical plan? And what was the prognosis?

The surgeon who asked John to walk in his office, who then had to catch him and tell him he'd never be normal again, was me. Before seeing him, I had read the report and checked the scan online when I was next in the office a day or two after receiving the referral, and so I had John come into my next open clinic. He told me and showed me that he couldn't open his clenched spastic fingers to hold a pen, or a knife and fork, or a wad of toilet paper. He could just manage to stand up on his wobbling spastic legs, but when he tried to step forward, his legs would cross — that scissoring is a sign of severe spinal cord dysfunction or myelopathy. It's another common syndrome in spine care, like sciatica.

The condition of disc bulges or bone spurs in the neck symptomatically compressing the spinal cord is called *cervical spondylotic myelopathy* (CSM). It's the most likely cause of acute neuromotor loss in an adult, and it's often quite painless — remember, pinched nerves (and spinal cords) don't hurt! Most commonly the early symptom is numbness. Some CSM patients will notice some loss of very fine motor control for a few months before the numbness sets in — their handwriting gets messy, or they have trouble texting or picking up their change from the counter at the coffee shop.

John's MRIs showed severe compression of the spinal cord at three disc levels, with one disc bulge in particular being quite massive. Likely that was what "blew out" when he fell. When spinal cords are acutely injured, they can cause terrible burning pain and extreme sensitivity to touch over the whole body, a condition called *allodynia*. We should all know what that is, we all get it for a few seconds after the blood rushes back into a numb foot. Imagine what it would be like if that feeling *didn't* go away when you stood and shook your foot for a few minutes, and if that feeling extended to your whole body!

Neurologically progressive (worsening) CSM is a surgical disease. There's no room for fiddling with pain meds or physio or injections at the pain clinic. It's critical to rescue that spinal cord as soon as possible, before it's too late!

How do we do the surgery? Depends on where the compression comes from, what the scan shows us and to some extent what the exact spinal cord injury syndrome is — there are several. Compression is most commonly anterior and we operate on the front of the neck, but when it's posterior we go from the back. Sometimes we might have to do both approaches!

Does the surgery work? Oh, yes. Some of the best current data we have on outcomes comes from the AO Spine group's prospective CSM cohort studies, and it tells us that 90 percent of patients will experience significant reversal of their neurological symptoms. Not usually *complete* reversal, and often leaving major deficits and disability, but major improvement.

How did it all work out for John?

The best predictor of how a surgical neurology patient is going to do is the condition of the patient coming into us. John was badly off. This was not a case for the waiting list. Neglectful care brought the patient to critical condition when surgery should absolutely have been done as soon as possible.

That's never easy in Canadian medical systems where hospital bed occupancy commonly runs over 100 percent. We virtually *never* have open beds for more than a few hours at a time despite hordes of dedicated administrators and managers doing their best to make it all work. So admitting John directly from the clinic was not a realistic option. But he *had* to be admitted. The actual surgery could realistically be accomplished without an inpatient stay if he'd been neurologically normal, but the degree of spinal cord injury and dysfunction meant he'd need some inpatient rehab too.

So I canceled somebody. Not the next week because everybody booked in that week was similarly critical, but somebody just a bit less urgent scheduled in the week after that. Never fun but sometimes necessary.

The surgery John needed for the disc prolapses in his neck — anterior cervical discectomy and fusion (ACDF) — is itself a modest thing. Cases involving just one or two discs are commonly done in private day-surgical suites without hospitalization at all! Canadian health practice doesn't allow for much of that, so we use the hospital, but even then, many of these operations will require only an overnight stay in the recovery room, and you're out and home the next morning. John wasn't the right patient for that because he was so badly off neurologically.

Surgery went great and he was much better as soon as he was awake enough to be evaluated in the recovery room. Better, but far from perfect. A dense neurological deficit such as John presented never recovers completely. There's usually a big improvement early on, but then it improves slowly and progressively, peaking at about a year.

A year later, he was walking without assistance but he was still slow and unsteady and awkward with all four limbs, lurching around my clinic with a cane. He'll never walk normally or do manual labor again.

All avoidable. Every time it happens. And I see it in my practice alone several times every year. A very real "spine crime": missed spinal cord compression and near paralysis. All for want of doctors asking a few simple questions of their patients and the common lack of spine care knowledge in the general medical field.

If you're not complaining about how sore or numb you are, your doctor might never know. So speak up and give them as much information as you can. And when there is something wrong, a good doctor asks you some questions about that: What hurts? Where are you numb? How did it start? Where and when are your symptoms worsened or relieved?

Doctors are innately programmed to save lives or prolong life, and many of our treatments can do that, in cardiovascular and cancer care for example. But most musculoskeletal and spine care doesn't save life at all; it addresses your aches and pains and treats your *quality* of life rather than its quantity. Although John's CSM and his terrible fall weren't fatal, his misdiagnosis made his life a living hell until he had the surgery he needed.

Many patients with spine-related neurological syndromes have very little pain at all, but some do. Most back pain complainants don't have surgical problems, and so doctors too often don't take them seriously or assess them well. We are effectively taught and encouraged to belittle back pain. "Get over it, you're not going to die from this."

Sometimes we're wrong.

Chapter 2

Horace the Dentist

He'd never leave his own patients' pain without proper care for weeks. Why did his doctors ignore his?

D entists work hard. They can be on their feet or bent over on a stool all day, peering into the mouths of people who often don't want the dentist to be there. Lots of stress in doing delicate technical work. It's no wonder their backs are sore and tired at the end of the day, never mind the week! My dentist patients tell me that over-the-counter (OTC) meds like Tylenol and Advil help them in their work a great deal, as do their chiropractors and massage therapists and physios.

Horace was one of those dentists. He did fine in his first decade of practice, but into his 40s, his back started getting sore regularly and he became one of the OTC crowd. He coped well and the practice flourished. Two assistants and several office staffers were kept busy and earned good salaries.

One late afternoon in his 48th year, the pain seemed different. It spread up towards his shoulder blades and burned a bit. No big deal, his usual remedies worked. At first.

This pain was odd. It didn't wax and wane. It was just there 24/7/365. Even lying down didn't relieve it. *Crap*, he later told me he'd thought, *middle age is a bitch.*

Then it got worse. Week to week to week. After a month, he was struggling with the workday, booking himself short and relying on his assistants a lot more than he was really happy with. One Saturday night he decided to cancel a dinner reservation he was too sore to enjoy and went to the ER to get checked out. The family doctor wasn't an option; hours there were Monday to Friday, which was when Horace was working at his own practice.

The ER was a madhouse. Horace arrived at 7:00 p.m. and didn't see the doctor until 11:30 p.m., a new guy just fresh into the night's work after the change of shift. Back pain? How long? Any numbness or tingling? No? Good. Any loss of bladder control? No? Better. Back sprain is common. Here's some Tylenol 3. Take it and go rest a bit.

Tylenol 3? Horace was a dentist. Many of his own patients needed more than that for their pain management! But what could he say? Sure, he'd try it.

ESCALATION

Tylenol 3 was garbage for this. He struggled through another abbreviated workweek and the next Friday was back at the ER. Waited again, three hours. The wiped-out day shift guy ordered an X-ray of his low back that another two hours later was reported to be perfectly normal, then he scribbled a prescription for some Percocet and ordered a CT scan of Horace's low back for the next week.

Percocet helped a bit. Horace could stand straight in the office but was tiring fast and always feeling cold, almost like the chills. Occasionally he'd have hot flashes and break out in a sweat, just for a few minutes. The scan happened on a Tuesday. Friday the family doctor called and told him it was fine and ordered more Percocet to be taken more often. He advised Horace that people got better pain control when they used their meds regularly rather than trying to tough it out until they couldn't stand it. Then he ordered an MRI to investigate further. CT scans are great for showing the bony anatomy but not so much for the soft flesh; maybe this was a disc or something.

The following Wednesday, work was a no-go. Horace dragged himself in but could barely stand — Percocet or not. He canceled all his patients and went straight to the ER at the large hospital near the office. He explained to the triage nurse and the ER doc that his pain was getting worse and worse and could they move up that MRI that wasn't scheduled yet? The ER guy laughed at that impossible thought, said hundreds of people were waiting for MRIs. He wrote up more Percocet when Horace refused a morphine prescription and tried to send the patient packing as quickly as possible. But when Horace started to yell in protest — he was in so much pain he wanted it dealt with once and for all and refused to be dismissed so easily — the ER doctor took off and ER Guy #2 showed up, apologized for his buddy and got on the phone to MRI. Sure, sure, we can do it at the end of the day.

Horace waited all afternoon, sitting in a hallway wheelchair because he couldn't stand and all the stretchers were full. Scan at 5:30 p.m., normal report at 8:00 p.m., and ER Guy #2 reappeared, now rumpled and tired and really grumpy towards the end of his shift. *He* yelled. Horace was told that he was another drug-seeking SOB, and the orderlies were called to throw him out of the ER when he refused to leave. They dragged him out of the place and he hobbled to his car. Managed to drive home, crawl into the house and crash out on the floor.

EXTREMES

Life on the floor wasn't bad; things hurt a lot less down there, but it was awkward at bathroom time. Forget showering. He made a lot of calls to keep the office going and didn't reveal his agony or embarrassment to anybody. All those ER guys said he'd get better quickly since the scans were normal, right?

Three days later a friend called, an ER doc at a small local hospital, and Horace broke down sobbing. The pain had continued to grow. Percs or not, his back was on fire, and even crawling around the house was hard. He'd had no urge to drag himself up onto the toilet all day and couldn't imagine doing that if he had. Ari came right over, took one look and called an ambulance to take Horace to his hospital's ER.

For the first time, in the quieter rural ER, the physician had a short conversation with his patient and asked a few simple questions. Nothing complicated. A big one was *Where does it hurt?* Horace painfully reached around behind himself and pointed towards the bottom of a shoulder blade. Another was *When did you last use the bathroom?* Yesterday. The ER doc did a bedside bladder ultrasound scan and immediately had her nurses insert a catheter to drain over a liter of urine out of Horace's bladder. A distended bladder or blocked flow of urine can cause fluid pressure to back up into the kidneys causing painful damage there, and that's on the differential diagnosis list of things that can cause problem back pain. When that didn't give Horace any relief, she ordered some spine X-rays that prompted an immediate emergency MRI scan. When that was done, she called the on-call spine surgeon.

WHAT WENT WRONG HERE?

No doctor likes back pain. In the majority, we don't understand it, get little formal training on it and generally can't do much about it. We commonly learn that most of these people seem to be looking for secondary gains like time off work or disability insurance money or drugs, so it's easy to make assumptions.

You'd think that the ER guys at the Big Hospital would be the best, and yes, they usually are. Most have years of specialty training and advanced qualifications to do what they do. That's great if you have an acute cardiovascular problem or major trauma or are morbidly ill needing resuscitation. Maybe not so much if you don't, or aren't.

None of the doctors at the Big Hospital took any history from this patient; nobody had any basic conversation at all. None of them read the triage nurses' notes after seeing the diagnosis "back pain." Nobody observed or examined Horace. They blew him off as a drug-seeking back pain complainant.

If they'd simply taken enough time to properly say "hello," they might have learned that this was a busy professional who'd never had problem back pain before and never taken a narcotic in his life. That he was disabled from his lucrative practice. That he could barely stand up!

That is not the profile of the gain-seeking back complainant. They are most commonly laborers or other workers with a long history of multiple recurrent back pain episodes associated with work or other heavy physical activity, never bad enough to limit normal daily activity and always better with the narcotics that they have typically been consuming for years.

If the Big Hospital staff had bothered to take any medical history, they'd have quickly learned a few key pieces of information:

1. This pain had come on spontaneously.
2. It was not relieved by rest.
3. It was rapidly growing in intensity despite increasing doses of powerful analgesics.
4. The pain was focused in Horace's mid-back, towards the shoulder blades.
5. There was a burning sensation associated with it (backache doesn't burn; neurological or neuropathic pain commonly does).
6. The patient was also feeling hot flashes and cold chills.

All of these things are classic red flags that should signal to the physician that something more important than common backache is going on.

WHAT HAD BEEN GOING ON FOR ALL THIS TIME?

At the Big Hospital, the ER doctors had assumed that Horace's back pain was a *low* back problem, the most common complaint, and so X-rays and scans of Horace's low back or lumbar spine had been done and were all normal. At the quieter Small Hospital, the ER physician who was less overwhelmed asked a few simple questions and immediately picked up two red flags suggesting a more serious problem than backache: Horace's pain was in the thoracic spine, up between the shoulder blades, and he hadn't passed urine in a day. Knowing the danger of untreated urinary retention, the scan and catheter were certainly the right things to do. When that didn't relieve his pain, she rightly ordered X-rays, not just of the kidneys (to check for kidney stones) but of the actual part of the spine that was painful — the thoracic spine. That simple X-ray, quick, cheap and immediately available, gave her the diagnosis — but she knew a specialist would need MRI info to plan care, so she had it done before making the referral. That urgent MRI scan was also properly focused at the thoracic spine.

There are 12 vertebrae in the thoracic spine, running from the low posterior base of your neck down to the top of the hollow of your low back. One for every rib. Horace's X-rays showed that the disc between T7 and T8 was missing, likely dissolved away by an infection, and that those two bones were collapsed down onto one another.

Just as cancers frequently spread to the bones of the spine when they metastasize, infections can spread to the spine — most commonly to the discs. As a student, I learned that this was a very rare thing, and in the global world of medical diagnoses it is, but it's always been known as a very important diagnosis because of the risk of paralysis. Every medical student is supposed to know to consider it in diagnosing problem back pain. Today this problem is increasingly common for unclear reasons. And yet two highly qualified ER doctors at the Big Hospital completely missed it.

The Small Hospital scan showed that what little remained of the T7/T8 disc was just a small wedge of liquid pus. A mid-thoracic disc like this is about an inch in diameter and a quarter inch tall. When it's abscessed, it basically becomes a giant zit squished between the adjacent bones. Remember having zits as a kid? No pain unless you were zapping them, right? In the spine, there's major pressure on the discs all the time, 24/7/365. That was Horace's early pain. It burned because the bulging disc pressed on the nerves alongside it.

In addition, without the cushioning disc separating them, physiological motion had the T7 and T8 bones rubbing on each other enough to actually be ground away in part. That's when it became difficult to support himself, and he had to lie down or recline in that ER wheelchair to take pressure off his spine.

The MRI scan showed that "the zit had popped"; the abscessed disc had ruptured and pus had been driven out into the spinal canal, compressing the spinal cord there. That's when Horace had suffered that last major spike in his pain, and spinal cord damage cost him the ability to control his bladder. Amazingly, somehow his legs still worked.

RESCUE SURGERY

I got the call just before midnight, a little after falling asleep at the end of a full day. *Shit.* We all need to rest. But this guy needed surgery, *now.* A rapidly deteriorating spinal cord is one of the few real spine care absolute emergencies.

I had him transported straight to my hospital's OR. Meanwhile, the OR called in an anesthesiologist and prepped out equipment.

When Horace arrived, his left leg was pretty darn weak. That was new and not good.

What surgery to do? Letting out the pus is a small thing. One simple laminectomy — a classical operation removing bone from the posterior (back) part of the spine bone (vertebra) to open the spinal canal and let out any pressure there — can often accomplish that. It's among the most elementary of spine surgeries.

But here the structure of the spine had been aggressively eroded. The patient's symptom history told me that, and it was confirmed in the OR even before the laminectomy was done. The spine was loose and wiggling all over the place as soon as it was exposed. That can't be ignored, every wiggle and wobble is stretching and twisting the delicate spinal cord. So this spine needed to be stabilized, or instrumented, with screws and rods too.

New problem. Surgical implants like to get infected, especially metals. That's a huge problem in hip and knee replacements. Not so much with spine implants for technical reasons, but no surgeon is happy setting hardware into a lake of pus.

In the wee hours of the morning, I could barely see straight much less think through details on how to address this vexing problem. What do you do when you can't do the case safely?

Change the game: the operation becomes a surgical care plan. There's a time-honored principle in orthopedic care that a problem bone infection may require several "cleanout" operations before it is safe to repair with implants. This is not a common practice in spine care but it makes good basic biological common sense, and so that's what I did. After surgically debriding (cleaning out) all the infection, I deposited antibiotic powder right in there, screwed the unstable spine together loosely and closed the wound.

A week later Horace was medically much better and in a lot less pain, despite the recent surgical wound. All his blood counts and biochemistry were stable or improving. Samples of pus taken at surgery had identified the infecting bacteria and what antibiotics it was most sensitive to. A special indwelling IV access catheter called a PICC had been inserted into his arm. He'd need IV antibiotics for months.

I took him back to the OR a second time just over a week later. After reopening the wound, I removed the potentially contaminated implant hardware I'd inserted at the first surgery and threw it all away. Then after thoroughly cleaning out the wound again, I reinstrumented with new sterile implants, "going long" to include several vertebrae both above and below the site of the infection to strengthen the fixation.

SURGICAL SUCCESS

The infection did well. Three months later, blood tests, X-rays and scans were all fine, with no evidence of ongoing infection at all, so the antibiotics were stopped and the PICC came out.

The spinal cord didn't do so well. Horace's left leg remained weak and spastic even after several months of inpatient spinal cord rehab, aggressive oral drug therapy and even after another operation where a pump had been inserted into the spine to flow spasm-breaking drugs right into the spinal fluid. Horace lurched around the house with a cane and needed a walker or a scooter to go outside for the rest of his life. He closed the office and had to put his staff out of their jobs. Luckily he had enough disability insurance to live on.

The bladder didn't do so well either, and Horace never passed urine normally again. For months he wore an indwelling Foley catheter inserted into his bladder through the penis and connected to a urine drainage bag attached to his leg. You can't do that forever because even the softest rubber catheter eventually erodes the delicate flesh of that organ, so in yet another operation a suprapubic catheter was inserted through his lower abdominal wall directly into the bladder. Every six months he was back to the day surgery for a catheter change because the things get clogged up all the time.

The patient didn't do so well either. Horace had trouble coming to grips with the drastic change in his life and saw a therapist for years. Five years after all this, he jumped off a bridge.

SPINE CRIMES

With great power comes great responsibility. No doctor should ever be too busy or too important to take a short history from their patient or to examine them a bit. If that had been done at the very first ER visit, or even by the family doctor before that, the red flags might have prompted an early scan of the correct part of the back. An early diagnosed disc infection commonly does well with a few months of IV antibiotics and that's that. Horace might have missed as little as a day or two from work, and his successful dental practice would still be thriving and employing people, looking after patients and paying a great deal of taxes. Most importantly, Horace would still have been here to tell the story.

Chapter 3
Frank the Trucker

It was just back pain. Most doctors
know that surgery's no good for that.
Sometimes they're wrong.

People like Frank are a common case at the pain clinic. Somehow a lot of men who are six and a half feet tall and 300 pounds end up driving trucks for a living. I don't know why that is. Both their size and the job are tough on their backs. Research going back to the 1990s shows the vibrations of a heavy engine accelerate disc degeneration, so surgeons like me see a lot of truckers in their 50s and 60s who have a long pain history and whose scans show their backs are shot.

These are the people who commonly give spine surgery a bad reputation among other doctors, mostly because spine surgeons can't do much for their pain unless it's associated with stenosis, deformity or instability — which it usually isn't. We don't see a lot of disabled truckers in their 30s though.

Frank was one of those. His job had been to drive a moving van, not long-haul work but a lot of loading and unloading. He was great at it for a decade until in his late 20s something went *pop* and that was it. Dropped the load he was carrying and never lifted another.

Burning pain in his low back, 24/7/365. Every move hurt. He had to spasm up all his core muscles to hold himself as stiffly as he could just to move around the house. No sciatica, no numbness or tingling or weakness in his legs. Just terrible back pain centered on his waistline.

THE STANDARD TREATMENT

No physician is happy to meet this guy. We've known for decades from research around the world that a physical worker injured on the job, someone who is on workers' compensation and is disabled for much more than a few months, has a very poor chance of recovering and getting back to work.

His family doctor suggested Tylenol and Advil together; when that didn't work, there were codeine and tramadol and antidepressants and nerve deadeners — and no benefit. Chiropractors couldn't get his odd twisty posture realigned. Physio? This guy couldn't exercise; he could barely move! At the pain clinic they injected his back with trigger point blocks and epidurals and facet blocks. Nothing.

When standard treatments fail, in many jurisdictions the compensation board sometimes takes things into its own hands and has the patient see the board's medical experts for comprehensive evaluation and treatment. In Frank's case, the neurologists said there was no neurology; the physiatrists (rehab doctors, nonsurgical physicians who commonly diagnose and treat neurological and musculoskeletal problems — and backache!) said he was too far gone for rehab; psychologists said he had chronic pain that would be permanent; the neurosurgeons and orthopedic surgeons said nothing could be done surgically. The board decided Frank would never work again and pensioned another "lazy-ass compensation freeloader" off for life. In his 30s!

I have yet to meet a disabled compensation patient who was living the high life on their small disability pension settlement. These people are commonly just barely getting by, leading a life of misery despite all the other social assistance options we have in Canada. A lot of those I meet use the food bank.

Frank was referred to a surgeon's office after begging his family doctor for the referral for over a year. His doctor said if the comp board says nothing can be done, then why bother?

Many surgeons like myself screen their referrals by looking over the MRI before accepting the consult. Why see patients whose scans don't show potentially surgical pathology? When I looked at this MRI it was interesting because, while the lowermost two discs were almost completely collapsed and worn out, the spine above them looked perfect. People who have worn out their spines from overwork usually have wear and tear everywhere. This fellow seemed different.

This great big man didn't have to stoop to get through the doorway of my office; his base posture was a forward bend of a good six inches or more. He shuffled around slowly, barely lifting his feet from the floor, wobbly but not using a cane. He did not look happy.

The medical history confirmed that his current pain had nothing to do with just doing work. It had been three years since his injury, and despite being off work he was in agony every day and every movement was painful. This man could barely dress himself and couldn't play with his young kids. He admitted to being suicidal sometimes.

Frank's pain was well localized to the lower back area. He didn't overreact to examination by screaming or crying out as so many chronic pain cases do. Muscle spasm extended across the whole length of his low back, up towards his shoulder blades and below his waistline to include the gluteus muscles of his buttocks, which were rock hard and a bit tender. Kinetically he was stiff as a board with every motion of the back. He could flex forward just enough to get his fingertips past his knees. *How does this guy put on a sock?* The muscles of his legs were strong. There was no sciatic nerve root irritation, and the reflexes were all normal. That's the classic profile of a write-him-off chronic pain complainant.

But a couple of things didn't fit. There are clinical signs we can find at examination called *Waddell's criteria* that help identify people who are hyper-reacting to their pain and therefore won't likely do well with painful surgery — he had none. Also, after bending forward as far as he could, Frank couldn't straighten back up properly because trying to do that caused his pain to spike.

He had to put his hands on his knees and walk his hands up his thighs to straighten. As he began to come up, a little after starting to straighten he'd flick his pelvis forward under his spine in what is classically called an *instability catch*, reversal of lumbar rhythm or Gowers's sign. And he never fully straightened, only came back to that baseline stoop he walked in with. With my hands on his chest and back I could gently drive him back towards a more erect position, but he flexed his hips and knees forward under him to accomplish it, and as soon as I let go he slumped forward again.

Clinically even at this point I knew he had an internal lumbar disc derangement (ILDD) and sagittal plane imbalance and that I could likely fix him.

WHAT DOES FRANK'S STRANGE KINETIC MOTION MEAN?

Let me explain something of how our discs work and why is it so easy to damage them. Be patient and hang in: it's going to take a few pages!

There are three joints between each of the vertebrae bones of your spine. The disc is in front (anterior, towards your belly) and the two bony facet joints are in the back. The neurological stuff is in the middle. The disc is the biggest of these three joints. They're something like a marshmallow with some jelly inside, or a jelly donut with no hole. Imagine squishing one of those between your fingers. You can see how the thing would be turgid (resist squishing) to provide support to the spine, and by rolling it between your fingers a bit you could understand how it might guide or direct motion somewhat. Those are the two major functions of a disc.

But discs are a lot tougher than marshmallows. They're more like a small hydraulic bushing or an engine mount. For you sports types, they might be compared to a golf ball or a baseball gone a bit soggy, with a very firm outer rim, or annulus, wrapped around a nucleus that's something like a jelly-filled water balloon. That nucleus is effectively overfilled with fluid and pressurized. When healthy, it has a colloid osmotic pressure of 1 to 3 atmospheres — and fluid cannot be compressed.

The healthy disc is actually stronger than the bone around it. When a young person has a high-impact injury, we don't find disc hernias — we find fractures, because the disc will act like a water hammer and rupture the bone around it.

Discs have to be that tough. They carry a load of three to four times one's body weight for several thousand load cycles every day, even with normal light daily activity such as bending or reaching. We load our spines something like four million times a year. No marshmallow's going to stand up to that!

Discs don't "slip out of place." If they're going to transfer those huge loads between vertebrae, they obviously have to be very strongly attached to them. And they are, through a thin connecting structure called an *end plate*. The end plate connection is incredibly strong. In the operating room, it's very hard to cut the disc away from the vertebrae with even the sharpest of surgical scalpels. When a disc hernia happens, only a very small piece of the disc generally moves out of place.

The healthy disc directs motion between the two vertebrae bracketing it. The "center of motion" was described by many, including a prominent Toronto surgeon from Sunnybrook Hospital named Stan Gertzbein way back in the 1980s. It isn't one perfectly fixed point but wobbles about just a bit, maybe a millimeter or two. So we can describe the spine below the neck as a column of 17 squarish bones, each balanced on a jelly donut sandwiched between them. A complex system of muscles and ligaments keeps it all aligned, balanced well enough to support your full body weight, and normally mobile.

If you've got a Fitbit or a health app on your smartphone, you likely know that in North America we average about 4,000 steps a day. The ideal for good health is 10,000. But every step is a load cycle compressing your discs. Squish squish squish on the jelly-ball annulus, bulge bulge bulge goes that compressed disc stretching against the annulus around it. The earliest anatomy of disc degeneration we can image is an inner rim tear of the annulus, likely caused by nuclear material pushing out against it. All the extension exercises and core strengthening that back pain patients are subjected to are really an attempt to stabilize these tears and stop them from enlarging. If they get big enough, nucleus material might start to migrate into them, get out to the edge of the annulus and rupture it and *bingo!* That's a disc hernia.

But when the tears are smaller and the nucleus can't move much, that "center of motion" can move just a bit out of joint. Likely a tiny bulge of nucleus is jammed into the inner annulus, stretching it but not enough to tear it. All of a sudden your spine is effectively partly dislocated, and in the same way a knee (or hip or ankle) with torn ligaments locks up rigidly in terrible pain as the body works to prevent further damage, the spine patient's core musculature locks up and they can't budge. That's an internal lumbar disc derangement (ILDD), an old diagnostic term I learned in the 1980s, which is not a common term in surgical spine diagnosis and care today.

Like everything, there's a spectrum of severity in ILDD, but a bad case is something like trying to walk around with a small sharp rock in your shoe. Every step hurts but if you limp and lurch just right, maybe you can still move around a bit without screaming.

When we lean forward, the support ligaments of our spine stretch out to carry more of the load. Bent forward fully at the waist, our muscles may be completely relaxed as the fully stretched ligaments support us. To straighten up from that bent position, we have to contract our back muscles to pull ourselves back up like a sailor pulling on the rigging to raise the mast of a boat. That contraction squishes the discs incrementally and will increase disc pressure and disc pain. So ILDD patients straighten up to a point and then flick their pelvis forward under their spine. That seems to let the spine take a more physiological "lordosis" posture that offloads the discs and makes it more comfortable to finish straightening up. To accomplish this, people often have to walk their hands up their thighs just like Frank did. Physiotherapists and knowledgeable doctors call it Gowers's sign.

WHAT CAN (AND DID) ALL THAT MUSCLE SPASM MEAN?

People will argue that all kinds of things can cause muscle spasm, and that's likely true. But when it's chronic and crosses the whole length of your back extending across to your buttocks, things may not be so simple.

There's a whole science today around the question of sagittal plane balance, meaning what the curves of your spine should be to allow you to stand and function normally. As our spines wear out, they can go out of alignment or "crooked" all kinds of ways, and that sagittal imbalance can be painful. Try it: lean forward for six inches or so next time you're going for a walk. Likely you won't be able to hold that position without pain for very long.

From standing X-rays, we can measure an alignment parameter in the pelvis called the *pelvic incidence* (PI) that predicts what the lumbar lordosis (LL) curvature should be. Ideally, they're within 10 degrees of each other (the arithmetic is PI-LL=10). LL commonly decreases with age as our discs dry up and shrink so PI-LL increases, and if it's more than 10, the patient is falling forward out of balance. Our bodies try to correct that with involuntary spasm of the back muscles hauling us backwards. This is likely a common reason for middle-aged backache at the end of the day. If that's not enough to get us up straight, then we rotate our pelvis backwards through spasm of the gluteus maximus muscle (that's your bum, people!). Rolling the pelvis back affects a third measure in those X-rays: pelvic tilt (PT). PT relates the base of your spine to the hips and they shouldn't be any more than about 20 degrees out of line either. If increased pelvic tilt can't get us balanced, we flex our hips and knees under us to assume a crouch gait, which is exactly what it sounds like: lurching around without ever fully straightening out hips and knees and ankles.

Smart spine surgeons today get standing X-rays on every new patient they see. I believe this should be a standard practice, and it is in fact recommended by some of the world's lead spine care societies. Frank's X-ray alignment was interesting: PI-LL>30, PT=30. This guy's lower two discs were so far collapsed that skeletally he was literally kinked forward about 20 degrees when he tried to stand up. He'd be in trouble from chronic muscle overstrain even without the kinetic ILDD problem.

SO WHAT TO DO ABOUT IT ALL?

When I started in practice over three decades ago, the treatment for a painful worn-out disc was to simply stabilize it. A fusion operation would create a solid mass of bone running between the vertebrae that bracketed the involved disc, taking motion and pressure off it. Back then we had no real knowledge of what the alignment should be and so a great deal of fusion surgery around the world left people out of alignment, or imbalanced. That's one of so many reasons why surgical spine care has its generally poor reputation; a lot of those people didn't do too well.

This guy needed to be both stabilized and realigned. There are several ways to do that, but basically two major variants.

We can operate through the belly to approach the affected discs directly and either fuse them or replace them with artificial discs (yes, that's a thing). There are three big problems with this approach to the disc. One, the biggest blood vessels we've got are plastered up against the front of the spine and it's not always easy to get them out of the way of our sharp cutting tools. Two, the fine nerves that control sexual function are right there and damage to them can make a male infertile, and a female numb. Last, it's very hard to dissect out this part of the spine in anybody who's the least bit heavy. So let's not.

We can operate through the back in a more traditional way. Some think that's easy, even in a big guy. Just feel back there and you're touching spine right away — how hard can it be? Not so easy. Even in smaller people there's often a good two inches of muscle between the skin and the spine, and in a large muscular man there can be three or four. That muscle has the texture of a raw roast beef (that's what roast beef is, the back muscle of a cow). So we have to cut through that with a minimum of muscle damage and without bleeding the patient to death, then we work our way into the spinal column itself and around the nerve sac to the collapsed discs under it. Then we clean out what's left of the disc material, jack up the collapsed discs to the right height, and implant spacers, commonly called *intervertebral cages*, and bone graft to the disc space to hold alignment and create fusion. Last, we have to screw it all together. All the while, our surgical tools are rubbing up against the great big nerve sac in front of us.

It takes easily five hours of patient-in-the-room OR time for me to reconstruct two discs on a normal-sized patient. This guy needed two more hours. Oh yeah, the extra time and work and stress are free; we surgeons are not compensated for complexity. That's another reason so many cases like Frank go untreated.

Almost eight hours in and out of the OR, a liter of blood loss. Practically killed me.

By the next morning Frank was better than he'd been in a decade, and he was walking comfortably that afternoon despite the great big cut. Catheter out the second morning after surgery, and home the day after that. Surgical pain of an open cut lasts about a month and Frank needed some mild narcotic pain meds for that long, as we'd expected. But then he stopped them. First time drug-free in almost four years.

Two months later Frank was playing with his kids again. Certainly he had some backache but so do most middle-aged people, including surgeons like me. At four months the silly fool was talking about going back to work and trying to hug his surgeon "thanks" in the office. He was allowed to go back to the job with some cautions, and he did . . . but only after long discussions with his employer's HR department and a meeting with his manager.

SPINE CRIMES

From an early age, Frank was on a long road to disaster and he was, and is, not alone. Many doctors and even surgeons commonly believe, teach and practice that back pain cannot be treated surgically. There are exceptions.

Chapter 4

Mike the Manager

A true tale of classic sciatica and why our
doctors need to know more.

T wenty-six years old, graduated with a management degree,
working in the successful family business. No wife, no kids, no
debt, no mortgage and bags of cash flow. Mike's life was *good*.

THE FIRST EPISODE

It all changed one typical day in the office when a client defaulted
on a loan and the file was in the bottom left drawer of Mike's desk.
When he leaned over to open the drawer, *Whap!* He felt a little
electric pop in his lower back.

He couldn't straighten up if his life depended on it because of
excruciating pain. The workday was over. He hobbled over to his
car, lay down in the back seat, and Dad drove him home.

A week later, the pain in his back was still there, work at the
office was backing up and the saga of care began. Advil and Tylenol
had been tested and proved useless by then, and stronger meds from
his family doctor didn't help much either. Wisely, Mike refused
narcotics. Tried some CBD oil, yuck.

Off to the chiropractor. The fellow announced that his patient had "put his sacroiliac joint out" and needed to have it manipulated back into place. That was going to take a series of at least a dozen fine adjustments and yes that's $75 bucks a visit, thank you. Where's your insurance card?

Ex-trauma surgeons like me learn from a cadaver experiment that one needs a 1.5-ton servo hydraulic testing rig to budge a sacro-iliac joint beyond its normal limits, so it's not likely that joint was injured reaching for a thin file of paperwork. And it's buried under several inches of fleshy muscle that has the consistency of raw roast beef. Nobody can feel a thing through that!

His chiro suggested massage might help too. That therapist gave a diagnosis of gluteal spasm and started stretching and rubbing that area. It only hurt a bit during the therapy and was a bit sore over-night afterwards. Same cost per visit.

After a few wasted months of all this, he was only just a bit better and still off work. Next, Mike was off to physio where he learned that the first two therapists were wrong. He had piriformis syndrome, a rare condition where the sciatic nerve is crushed by an abnormal piriformis muscle at the hip. This could also be treated, with piriformis stretching and ultrasound, to the tune of $60 a visit three times a week.

A smart person might think to ask, Why didn't this abnormal muscle hurt for the first 26 years of Mike's life? Most people in pain can't or don't think that much, so they let their insurance pay the bills while they wait things out.

Six weeks later Mike's pain was pretty much settled and he was back at work part-time when the appointment for an MRI his family doctor had ordered on day one finally came up. The report said he had a bulge in the lowermost disc of his back that could be causing sciatica. His doctor wanted to refer to a surgeon but Mike didn't want that. After four months of pain and therapies he was finally getting better in a big way, so why have surgery? He opted to delay and a month later was working full time.

Disc bulges are extremely common. Population research studies have consistently showed that the odds of a random scan revealing one in an asymptomatic patient are roughly equivalent to our age in years. Most don't cause any sciatic trouble because they're not big enough to impact the sciatic nerve roots; they just harmlessly bulge into the spinal fluid bath. But when Mike leaned over sideways to reach into that left bottom drawer of his desk, the loads on his lower discs skyrocketed and he ruptured one!

The nerve roots from the low back link up to form the sciatic — and femoral (whatzzat? more later) — nerves alongside the lumbar spine. The sciatic nerve then goes downward on each side through the posterior abdomen to exit the pelvis through a bony structure called the *greater sciatic notch*, and then run down the back of the thigh towards the foot. That bony notch is just underneath your butt muscle (or *deep to* your butt, as we medical types describe it). Because the sciatic nerve doesn't connect to many major sensory nerve endings in your back, the inflamed nerve itself can become tender and that pain locates to where the nerve comes out of the pelvis, close to the surface of the posterior upper thigh just at the bottom of the buttock. So, sciatic pain is quite literally a pain in the ass!

I wish every doctor knew that.

Reader, here's a thing. Having sciatica doesn't mean you have a disc hernia. Sciatica is a symptom that can be caused by many different things compressing the nerve or its roots. As we will learn as you read along.

As a student, I learned decades ago that acute back or sciatic pain episodes almost always resolve themselves quite quickly, most in a few weeks and some in a few months. The body's natural inflammatory reactive biology causes the disc bulge to resorb — even without any treatment at all! This doesn't happen quickly. It's a gradual process that extends over several months — but when it does unfold this way the patient usually notices improvement within the first few weeks, and then month to month for three or six months they're getting better and better.

So, we could apply almost any kind of treatment in that situation and it would seem to work. All the drug and physical therapies available can justify themselves for early pain relief on this basis, but sadly just about none are shown to change where your back is going to be six months or a year or two or five or 10 down the line. A large quantity of good-quality research that focuses on acute episodes like this supports all the treatments out there, and so nonoperative therapy has become a huge business around the world. I make a bad joke with the rare acute-care patients I see that I could lock them in a purple-painted room with a flashing yellow light and charge them for that psychedelic experience, and in the majority they'd get better and love me for it — and they likely would!

It is now common for spine surgeons with an interest in providing primary, or acute, spine care to affiliate with rehab clinics of various sorts. Allegedly we are practicing good care by referring these cases to rehab to try to avoid surgery, but too often the reasons may be financial, as surgeons undertake to cash in on the business of rehab like everybody else does.

When Mike bulged his disc the first time, it wasn't big enough to cause sciatica running down his leg, but it did irritate his nerve enough to cause sciatic pain. The nerve's location is only an inch or so from the sacroiliac joint, alongside it, and that same distance above the piriformis muscle. When structures are deep enough in the flesh that you can't really feel them with any accuracy, it's easy to mislabel sciatic pain as these other things.

I'd say sacroiliac joint pain is a myth. Sadly today it's being played up aggressively in the spine surgical world, largely driven by one company that brought out an appealing minimally invasive surgical (MIS) technology for sacroiliac fusion a few years ago.

Massage therapists call this sciatic notch tenderness gluteal spasm, and in fact those muscles may spasm in this condition. But spasm in the spine is almost always a *reactive* phenomenon. It's the body trying to protect itself from injury rather than an injury unto itself. Prolonged spasm can itself cause muscle pain, and anybody who's ever overdone it at the gym knows that. Massage is just one of the many counter-irritant therapies that can temporarily relax muscle spasm. So the sciatic patient commonly gets some massage — and it works: a few weeks later they're somewhat better (just like they would likely have been without it!).

THE SECOND EPISODE

What I as a student wasn't taught about all those patients with acute disabling spine conditions that usually get better was that about 10 percent of those patients go on to have multiple further similar episodes, and *that* population really never settles down completely. We don't often know *why* they have these further episodes, only that they do. I think it's likely that they continuously reinjure themselves. People and their caregivers, medical or otherwise, in the majority, don't really understand the back well enough to explain it to people, and even for you the patient it's back there behind you — out of sight is out of mind and before you know it — *ouch!*

We understand our sprained ankle (or most other injuries) easily enough. It's there on the end of our leg in front of our eyes, purple and swollen up twice as big as the other one. Any idiot knows to take it easy on that ankle. We may not put weight on it for weeks, and after a few months we forget about it enough to run for a bus or stop babying it at the gym. We don't "burn in" that kind of image with a back injury and so in no time flat — bend, twist, recurrent pain!

Neither the chiro, the massage therapist nor the physio actually *gave* Mike any elementary education in spine mechanics or the importance of good posture. When his surgeon later explained some elementary mechanics, he was amazed and a bit upset that he had never been given that simple information earlier. They'd all simply taken his insurance company's money. A lot of it.

So sure enough, a few months after recovery, Mike was lifting his expensive golf clubs into the trunk of his car, and when he leaned forward to gently put them down — *pop!* His back was "out" again.

This time it was worse. The pain was much more intense, burning down the back of his leg across the calf onto the heel, sole and outer edge of his foot. He limped, stooped forward and had to lean to the side away from his sore leg even to hobble around the house. The only way he got some relief was lying on the floor with his legs propped up on a chair, bent at the knee. He couldn't lie down in bed and had to sleep sitting up curled in a ball on the edge of the sofa.

For nine months. Off work. While the chiro and massage and physiotherapists did their thing again. Uselessly this time.

Remember earlier I said most disc hernias get better by hand of God? That's true. *Most* means roughly three out of four. For reasons we often don't completely understand, roughly one in four just doesn't settle down, or it does and then recurs and might qualify for surgery.

What qualifies a disc for surgery? No, not just a good health insurance plan and an available operating room! Rarely, patients might have uncontrollable pain or a major neurological deficit, that's obvious. Most commonly we might operate for intolerable symptoms (commonly, pain and/or neurological deficit) that (1) have been present for more than a few months (my teachers used to say, "Never operate before three months because the disc may settle down by itself" — like Mike's did at the first episode); that (2) cause pain that is not controlled by medicines, not settling down or perhaps even getting worse; and (3) that are bringing an unacceptable disability to the patient.

This last point is key — I feel strongly that the unique risks of surgery should only be lined up against disability, not irritating symptoms. Lots of people have sciatic syndromes they can live with. In the majority we don't expect them to get worse and worse or to paralyze anybody. If the patient can live with it, so should the surgeon. Research studies consistently show that with disc hernia, 10 years later one is not much better with the surgery than without it. Sciatic disc surgery is really for a short-term gain, for immediate relief of symptoms and disability.

Disability is a very subjective thing. I've had people limping around on a cane who could live with that, who had worked out a tolerable and acceptable lifestyle around it and never came to surgery. And I've had people who were slowed down just a bit in their favorite sports and couldn't live with that. Up to them, as long as the risks of surgery are clearly explained when the time comes. Even today's oh-so-fashionable minimally invasive surgery can injure or kill the patient — and yes, that actually happens.

DEALING WITH IT

Mike wasn't a complainer and in a lot of ways didn't have to be because of his privileged situation in life. He wasn't laid off from his job for sickness because it was the family business, and so his bills were still paid. That doesn't happen for most people. I treat spine care patients all the time who have lost the house, and sometimes the spouse, over this kind of situation.

After six months or so Mike asked his family doctor for another scan and it showed his disc bulge was still there and even bigger that it had been at first. His doctor referred him to a surgeon.

His surgeon flipped out a bit when they met. Here was an otherwise fit young man who'd been disabled for nine months and troubled for almost two years by a simple disc bulge. Shouldn't happen in any reasonable modern health care system. Discectomy surgery, where we remove the bulge to unpinch your nerve roots and relieve sciatica, has been standard spine care since 1934 and it virtually always works well for the sciatica patient with a disc hernia. It's been day surgery for several decades (I published on it, in a small way, way back in 1999). It takes about an hour to do these operations, though we usually have to book two hours of OR time to allow for equipment processing and turnover and whatnot.

After two hours in an operating room Mike woke up without sciatica for the first time in two years. Later in the day he went home to sleep comfortably in his own bed — lying down flat!

Two weeks later at the clinic he was standing straight and not limping. He was taught some very simple isometric back-strengthening exercises, to help regain basic fitness that he had lost through two years of inactivity.

Six weeks later at the surgeon's office he was pain free, working full time and wanting back on the golf course. The surgeon said no because of the bending and twisting that come with that sport; after surgery many of us like to hold people back from such activity for three months.

His surgeon never saw him again and didn't want to. Good health care relieves the problem and returns the patient to their lives, making room for the next case.

SPINE CRIMES

Nine months of needless recurrent sciatic disability in any modern health care system is a spine crime. This guy was lucky he didn't lose his job or his house. What happens when someone like this has a family, young kids? What's the impact on a relationship, on the kids watching Dad limp and lie around and no-I-can't-play-with-you, listening to Mom upset about bills not being paid and thinking maybe Mom and Dad are breaking up because they can't sleep together in the same bed anymore? Lives are ruined by the effects of simple but real back ailments — not just the patient's life, but the whole family's.

Mike should have been scanned and referred not with his first episode but no later than three months into his second, and likely right away then because his symptoms and disability were so bad.

In similar circumstance, you all should be. Your doctors should all know that. And your physiotherapists and chiropractors and massage therapists and osteopaths and reflexologists and pain clinic doctors and everybody else involved in the spine care business should too. Too many don't.

Chapter 5
Mary the PSW

Worse off with spinal stenosis than most of her patients.

Home care support for the ill and elderly is commonly provided by professional personal support workers, PSWs. The work of a PSW isn't easy. Drive to the client's home, help them bathe or change their wound dressings or even feed and clothe them. Old, sick, weak people who can often barely move. This is very physical work. And it's stressful time-challenged work — do it wrong and people could get sick or be hurt. And watch the clock because if you spend too much time with one client, you may not have enough time to look after the next. Drive fast but don't speed, in and out of the car and up and down a zillion different sets of stairs with all that gear. Sheesh.

In her early 50s, Mary was just a few years short of the meager pension that followed the lousy salary. Backache? Geez, backache started just a few years into the job, and it's just a part of that life, nothing to complain about. Middle age is a bitch. Stuff hurts! But that hip. Man oh man! A deep searing ache started in her right hip just after her half-century birthday and slowly got worse with the years; not much change from month to month but year to year it was stronger and more sore. At 53 it was zinging down through Mary's leg and at 54 she was limping at the end of the day. Over-the-counter meds from the pharmacy and glucosamine from Costco didn't help at all, so with reluctance she complained to her family doctor.

AT THE DOCTOR

After listening to Mary's hip pain complaint her doctor suggested she try blah blah blah blah blah from the pharmacy counter. Oh, what, did that already? Gee, maybe it's something serious, let's get an X-ray.

The X-ray report was normal so it was time for physio. Two thousand dollars' worth of physiotherapy later, Mary's employee benefits were exhausted but her leg was heavier and starting to feel like she was dragging it around at the end of the day.

Try some arthritis medicine until we get an ultrasound test for bursitis. Normal.

Try some mild narcotics until we get an MRI of your hip. Normal.

Oh, your pain's chronic, now try an antidepressant. No? Well now there's medical marijuana available, try that . . .

With a mortgage to pay, giving up her job was not an option, so Mary kept at it but otherwise cut her usual activity back to the point where she was ordering all her groceries online and wasn't seeing friends. All she could do at the end of the day was limp around the house a bit. Her marriage was strained.

She'd been to the family doctor a dozen times. With all the test results being normal, there was nothing to offer, and she was added to the two-year wait list for the chronic pain clinic after the doctor grilled her about her life and her marriage and made sure she wasn't being abused, because pain can be psychological.

Late one evening as she hobbled down the stairs at home, her leg buckled under her and down she went like a bag of cement. Her hip pain spiked intensely; she couldn't move much less get up. That's it, said her husband, let's get you to the ER.

At the ER a nurse took her story and she had a hip X-ray done that was as normal as the first that her family doctor had ordered. After a sleepless night, she met a nice young man from the internal medicine service (What's that?) who listened intently for a half hour, taking copious notes as she told her story, and then announced that she was being admitted for a diagnostic workup (What's that?).

She just about couldn't move in the ward bed, her intense, deep burning pain spiked with the least motion and using the bedpan was torture. She soiled herself a lot because the nurses couldn't help her fast enough and she began to appreciate what good service she had been giving her own clients through the years. If she could get a team of her buddies in this place, they'd clean it right up!

More drugs every day; different drugs every day because nothing worked. She learned that with enough morphine on board, it was true, you did slur your words and see double. But you could still hurt!

Consultant after consultant after consultant. Orthopedics. Rheumatology. Neurology. Eventually the hospital-based pain service, who offered to inject drugs right into the hip where the pain was coming from — *please!* Two hours on an ice-cold fluoroscopy table in the pain clinic and the needle was finally in the right place . . . but nothing happened. Her "frozen" hip still hurt.

Next morning the pain service doctor consulted with Medicine and suggested that maybe just maybe this wasn't hip pain after all; maybe it was something else. Spine pain is common; we do injections for that all the time! It was agreed they would try and get an MRI scan of her back as soon as possible. More visits to that pain clinic torture chamber. Epidural steroids, not once but three times? Sacroiliac blocks. Facet blocks. Nothing helped.

Mary's MRI finally made a diagnosis. Spinal stenosis — that's a surgical disease but a treatable one. A consult was called out to the spine service.

On the medical ward at midday, Mary was asleep. When the consultant spine surgeon woke her up she was obviously stoned. The morphine dose was so high her pupils were contracted down to nothing and she was heavily sedated. That's a dangerous thing in itself: too much narcotic sedation and you stop breathing. You can die. So the consultant knew that she had to write down the dosing of the patient's drugs and to do something here.

Once Mary was conscious she was an obvious mass of pain and wouldn't move in the bed. There were early bedsores on her heels after being largely motionless for three weeks. She was asked to take a finger and point to where it hurt and she called the lady an idiot, *WTF don't you know where the hip is?* She asked again and Mary pointed to her buttock with a trembling index finger before dozing off again. Bingo! Your hip is nowhere near your buttock.

Anatomically the hip is just deep to the inner/medial groin at the top of your thigh and that's where hip pain is located. The buttock, now *that's* where sciatic pains locate. None of the allegedly qualified physicians who had been seeing and treating Mary for three weeks even knew where a sore hip should hurt!

Mary couldn't even be examined properly because she was in too much pain. Just to touch her leg brought a yelp and tears. She could wiggle her toes and ankle a bit but that was it; any attempt to lift her leg or bend at the hip or knee brought a scream of pain. Her leg muscles were not shriveled and she could feel a light touch on her leg, but that was all that could be done for a neurological exam. Mary couldn't contract her leg muscles forcefully at all because of pain when she'd try. There were good pulses in her feet so the doctor knew this wasn't a blockage of the circulation, another common cause of severe pain and motor strength loss in the leg.

The MRI showed that she had severe spinal stenosis at several disc levels in her low back. Disc degeneration and spinal stenosis most commonly affect the lowermost two discs, what we call L4/

L5 and L5/S1. Although those two discs were worn out, dried up and badly collapsed, they weren't bulging and the nerves were not pinched. But at each of the next three levels, going from L1 to L4, they were.

From the cross-linking of our sciatic nerve roots alongside the spine comes not just one nerve (the sciatic) but two. The lesser of these is the femoral nerve that connects to the anterior thigh from the groin down to the knee. The nerve roots affected there don't run to your feet and ankles to cause drop foot and stumbling, as in common sciatica. They go to the bigger stabilizing muscles at your hip and knee, the muscles that brace your leg out straight to take your weight when you stand. Here we had *three* points of compression. This lady wouldn't have had the strength to stand even if her pain *were* controlled! I honestly don't think the doctors Mary had previously seen knew that basic anatomy.

After three weeks in hospital the menu of pain care options had been pretty well exhausted and really there wasn't anything left to offer her other than surgery, which involved cutting away the bulged discs and bone spurs to unpinch her nerves. Generally, that can be a very small operation easily accomplished as a day procedure or at most an overnight stay, but Mary's bedridden clinical condition argued for inpatient care. After the surgeon explained the procedure, Mary accepted and gave consent, and she was put on the operating room's "add board" list where urgent cases line up to wait for care. Usually things get done within a few days. In Canada, the doctor can't just snap his fingers and have an operating room immediately available like they do on TV.

Days? she asked. *What do you mean, days? I'm dying here Doc!!! Do something!*

The surgeon had one last trick to try. Long ago it was common to give oral steroids for acute sciatica, and in the States there's something called a *Medrol dose pack* (marketed for rheumatoid arthritis flareups) that is used similarly. It's now considered an unorthodox practice and there's not a lot of published literature on it, for no good reason other than oral steroids are dirt cheap and there's no money to be made with that research. (Around the world there's a roaring "pain clinic" business injecting steroids all over the spine. Big bucks there, but not with oral drugs.)

As a last-ditch attempt to ease her suffering quickly, the surgeon offered Mary the oral steroids prescription, adding that these were powerful drugs and the side effects could be enough that she might not tolerate them. She was willing to try.

PLANS FOR SURGERY

Mary's name came up on the OR list four days later, and the OR couldn't find her! After several phone calls, it became apparent that the steroids had worked so well that she had been able to get up and move around a bit with a walker and took herself home! Pretty good, eh?

The surgeon called her into the office a week later to see what was up. Mary was getting around a bit and much more comfortable with the steroids on board, but she was still in pain and still not very mobile. She very much wanted the operation and was booked for a simple decompression a short while later. But when the surgeon brought up her imaging on the OR computer she had the scare of her life!

Wise surgeons get standing X-rays done on new low back consults. Spines can reveal a lot under gravity that's hidden when we're lying down, as on a standard X-ray table (or in the MRI scanner). Standing X-rays are standard practice in deformity surgery like scoliosis but not common in simpler surgeries, for no good reason really. Historically the patient lies down for imaging of most body parts and that's just the tradition. Those standing X-rays had not been done on Mary when she was first seen because she was simply too sore to stand up, but she'd had them done now in pre-op and *wow* did her spine collapse under gravity. Compared to her lying-down (or supine) X-rays, when standing up, she collapsed sideways into a scoliosis that shifted her whole trunk off to the left by an inch! Every single disc in her back had collapsed to bone-on-bone such that, from a side view, she was bent forward through 40 degrees rather than exhibiting the normal-looking lumbar lordosis curvature of the low back, which arches backward. No wonder she couldn't stand or walk much!

Doing just a decompression on a case like this would be a disaster. When we trim away arthritic bone spurs to unpinch the nerves, we are effectively removing some of your spine's support structure. There's always some risk we might remove too much, in which case the spine can painfully collapse and need a structurally reinforcing instrumentation and fusion operation (that is, fusion of the vertebrae and insertion of rods and screws). If the spine's already collapsing (unstable) to start with, like Mary's, reconstruction is essential.

Mary's spine would need stabilization across the whole length of her low back, from T10 to pelvis, which in English pretty much means bra line to bum, and you can't do that safely in just a few hours. It takes the better part of a whole OR day.

Back at the bedside, the surgeon explained the X-ray findings and what they meant, canceled the decompression surgery with an apology and scheduled Mary back into the office the next week to explain things again, show her the films and update the consent for the bigger operation this problem needed.

Mary was OK with all this. Nobody wants to have the wrong operation, and this was a narrow escape for both surgeon and patient. A month or so later they were back for a loooong day in the OR; the surgery took nine solid hours to accomplish.

Mary recovered well and spent six months avoiding bending of the body (to protect her screws as the fusion healed) and then gently exercising to get her strength back. At the one-year post-op visit she had some mild backache but no disability, no "hip pain" and was back to her normal life. With no pain there was no back muscle spasm and so her body could stretch and move *around* her spine, mostly through the hips. She could even touch her toes.

Although Mary was feeling much better, she decided to retire. All those years as a PSW had taken a huge toll and she now wanted to concentrate on looking after herself. Smart move!

SPINE CRIMES

It takes very little not just to ask but to have the patient *show* the doctor where it actually hurts. Doctors are just about never taught to do that, and it commonly leads to misdiagnosis — and worse, to having the wrong surgery — out of ignorance.

I've operated on all kinds of people who have had ineffective joint replacement surgery, for the sin of their hip or knee X-rays showing common middle-aged wear-and-tear degeneration, when they really had a neurological compression. And vice versa! Just the day before doing an edit on this chapter, I saw a man who'd been referred by not one but two — *two* — different orthopedic surgeons, both having diagnosed sciatica when it turned out that his pain came from bone-on-bone arthritis at the hip. In Mary's case, once the real problem had been diagnosed, pure blind luck saved her from the disaster of having the wrong spine surgery.

Mary got doubly lucky here. And didn't need a malpractice lawyer like Larry . . .

Chapter 6

Larry the Lawyer

Who lost his own case to cancer.

Larry was a very successful lawyer. Or not.

Straight from undergrad to a top law school, he graduated near the top of his class after being headhunted for articling in his first year. He passed the bar in his sleep and was bringing in big bucks in financial and malpractice law right off the bat. Being tall and good-looking didn't hurt. The opposition was intimidated and the ladies . . . oh the ladies . . .

Wife #1 was OK but pregnant way too fast and way too often, #2 was more fun but young and stupid, #3 was a professional match but he didn't like her challenge and so she was gone quickly too.

In his mid-50s he was flying solo and living large, had a hot Jag parked at his luxury downtown condo, and who needs a wife with the Internet dating apps we have today? We could all hate this guy. He didn't even get a middle-age spread and stayed trim no matter how little he hit the gym.

Court trials can be tough, lots of stress and you can be up on your feet for hours. Approaching middle age, some backache is common. The gym helps, some Tylenol in your suit pocket helps, even vodka helps.

One day at the gym Larry pulled something in his upper back. Wasn't too bad, he powered through his workout and racked up 11 billing hours that day besides.

A week later it still hurt. Tylenol.

A week later it still hurt. No gym.

A week later it still hurt. Advil.

A week later it still hurt. A doctor visit. Percocet.

A week later it still hurt. More Percocet. Hard to stand up for very long. No court, no office.

A week later it still hurt. A hospital visit. Really hard to stand up despite the Percocet.

Larry was admitted to the internal medicine service of the hospital for a diagnostic workup. Had a bunch of blood tests, CT and nuclear medicine and MRI scans of his low back. They were all fine. All the while his pain was getting stronger and stronger and stronger, and he felt weaker and weaker and weaker.

After two weeks of this, he was pretty much bedridden. A neurology consultant didn't find much. The pain service jacked up his meds, the Fentanyl patches helped, so he could move around a bit — for a week. Then a physiatry consultant said he could be helped with inpatient rehab care; obviously he was too weak and "deconditioned" to go home.

Every week in the hospital the attending doctor was a new guy, a common thing for inpatient medical care in some teaching hospitals. He didn't see much of the week one and week two people, but the week three guy said they should scan him again before sending him off to rehab, just in case. He ordered a whole spine MRI.

Short of certain specific indications, many surgeons hate whole spine MRIs because they suggest that nobody has either examined the patient or knows what they're doing. It's a fishing expedition. Also, false positive MRIs in middle-aged and older people may be more common than not. These scans find a great deal of degenerative change and even neurological impingements that don't bother the patient at all and so don't warrant care.

But not always.

Larry's scan showed a large cancerous tumor in his thoracic spine, his upper back between the shoulder blades. It had eroded the bone a little bit but most of the structure was intact and the alignment was preserved, so nothing looked unstable and that was good. The bad thing was that it had grown into his spinal canal and had compressed the spinal cord aggressively. That's why he was lying still in the bed while the doctor told him all this bad news — even rolling over in bed hurt!

And you know, the bed smelled like piss — *Why can't the damn nurses clean it up?* By this point he was too weak to get up to the bathroom, and he'd try to hold it till they brought a bedpan but too often he couldn't.

Doc, that's where my back has been hurting all along! Why didn't this show up in the earlier scans?

The doctor was surprised that nobody had asked him that important little question, *Where does it hurt?* He explained that all the earlier scans had been focused on his low back where problems are most common. No apology. He said he'd call a spine surgeon to operate on him, have the nurses insert a bladder catheter to stop the bedwetting problem, and left.

A nurse came in and put the catheter in. Larry thought it would hurt but it didn't; actually he didn't feel a thing. *Couldn't* feel a thing down there. When it was done, the nurse squatted down beside the bed to see how much urine had emptied into the collecting bag. She stayed down there a long time. Got up with a worried expression and her eyes all big and round, went off to get a bedpan and emptied the bag into it. Stayed down there again for a while afterwards. Larry learned that there was almost a liter and a half of urine in there. That's several times more than most people can hold in their bladder and enough to cause serious back-pressure damage to the bladder muscle and even the kidneys.

A little while later, a spine surgeon showed up to talk to him. He explained that there was a cancer in his spine crushing the spinal cord, likely a metastatic cancer that had spread there from some-where else. Finding the primary site would take some time; Larry would need a whack of further testing. But regardless, because the spinal cord was crushed and he was becoming paralyzed, the thing to do would be an operation to remove the tumor from his spinal cord in the hope that his paralysis would reverse, and that he'd get some if not most of his strength back.

The surgeon explained that this was a big deal: tumors can bleed a lot and he'd likely need transfusions and screws inserted in his back during surgery. But it was a great operation to alleviate pain and disability. Apparently things called *outcomes research* and *QALY analysis* suggested that the single most effective thing that can be done in health care is metastatic spine care, not cardiac surgery or anything else. The surgeon also explained that spine surgery can't cure cancer. When it was over, Larry would still need radiation treatments and chemo and God knows what else.

Larry by this point had been Larry the Patient for way too long. He was a shriveled paralyzed wreck of a guy, but his brain still worked despite all the narcotics and Larry the Lawyer was still in there. He wasn't an idiot despite looking (and smelling) like a salvaged street person. So he asked the obvious question.

What about this little paralysis problem, Doc? It's such a great operation for pain, but will I get my legs and bladder function back?

No promises. The surgeon told him that across-the-board outcomes research showed that roughly 70 percent of thoroughly decompressed metastatic paralysis cases would get "major improve-ment" of their deficits. Major improvement. Not complete reversal. In Larry's situation, with a dense paralysis and a paralyzed bladder, at this point the odds of standing and walking anywhere close to normally were just about zilch. Post-surgery, he'd likely be in a wheelchair forever, and the bladder function only rarely returns.

Nobody's a courtroom star or the office stallion from a wheelchair with a catheter bag attached to it. No Jag without hand controls, if they even make them. No babes. Larry's charmed life was over.

What if we picked this up a month ago, Doc, would I still be paralyzed? Likely not. He'd still have been needing all the cancer care but he would have been neurologically intact at the time of diagnosis. He might have gotten away with just a needle-stick percutaneous biopsy to confirm the diagnosis, and if his cancer was sensitive to radiation or chemo, he might not have needed any surgery at all. He might have done well for a long time. Metastatic spine care cases across the board live for an average of about two years, and depending on the type of tumor sometimes for decades.

Heyyy . . . Larry the Lawyer had a fleeting thought. *Bastard docs had me in here all month and let this happen to me, big cash in that lawsuit. Money in the bank!*

But so what, he'd still be driving a wheelchair. And likely smelling like pee. Not an attractive lifestyle. Larry was angry and fed up. He wasn't having any of it — what for, a couple of years of misery and chemotherapy poisoning?

When he said *No,* to the surgeon, the guy responded, *What do you mean, no? Surgery is the best treatment for this! You have to have the surgery, otherwise there's no hope.* He was almost desperate.

Larry the Lawyer smelled trouble in that desperation. *Did the guy need to feel so bad? And for what?* Larry the Lawyer could be a Rude Dude, and when he bluntly challenged his surgeon this way the guy paled — and then Larry saw the medical doctor peeking into the room through the doorway and understood the CYA (Cover Your Ass) that was going on. Larry said a few more choice rude things to them both, and they left.

They never came back.

A day later an oncology doctor showed up and explained the process of workup that would allow Larry's health care team to firm up the cancer diagnosis. Oh goody, now Larry had a health care team — where'd they been for the last month? And don't these clowns even talk to one another? This "team leader" didn't seem to know that Larry had decided against further care, so Larry told him to get lost.

A few days after that, a palliative care doctor came by and explained all the wonderful things that could be done to ease his pain and support his care when he would be transferred to the palliative care unit. It would take at least a few days to get a bed there, maybe a week. Interesting concept, but why take pain meds? By this point Larry had no pain. Simply couldn't feel a thing below his shoulders. Smelled better than he had in a long time. That catheter had been a good idea.

Three weeks later, unnoticed and alone, Larry just quietly stopped breathing one night. Nurses found him cold in the morning. Fortunately he had signed a "no code" form beforehand so nobody tried to resuscitate him. Two hours later there was another fully insured patient in his bed.

SPINE CRIMES

Terminal paralysis from unrecognized cancer missed by multiple caregivers and even in a patient who has been hospitalized. All for want of anybody simply taking a few seconds to ask exactly where it hurts.

It's not all just about backache, folks.

Chapter 7

Samantha's Sore Feet

Spinal cord surgery can be big, long and grueling — and so can the fallout from not doing enough of it.

For a lot of people, life is very tough. Poverty, broken families, lax or lacking education. These are often both the neediest and most resilient people in our world. When you have nothing and know little and have few supports, you've got to have something inside yourself that keeps you going. You've got to be tough and a bit stoic. But it is possible to be too tough and stoic . . .

A TOUGH CASE

In her late 30s, Samantha had survived it all and was well on the way to turning her life around. She'd quit smoking two years earlier and had begun taking long walks every day for at least an hour each, two walks some days. She felt pretty good for it all. She'd not worked much in that time, but social services disability support was enough for a small clean apartment that she shared with her daughter as well as groceries and a cheap cellphone plan.

In the spring and summer, she liked to wear sandals, and oddly one year, she'd noticed her feet getting cold during her walks. They didn't swell or turn colors or feel numb or anything — they just got cold a lot. So she took to wearing her runners even in warm weather.

Through the fall her feet always felt cool so she wore thick socks all the time, even in the apartment. She mentioned her cold feet to the doctor when she was getting her diabetes medicines renewed one day, and when the doctor examined her feet she said everything was fine there: strong pulses and no varicose veins or swelling and Sam could feel everything the doctor touched so no nerve damage. Wear some socks!

Samantha didn't tell the doctor that her feet were starting to feel heavy too. Increasingly she would stumble at home, and she took more and more to shuffling around the place. That wore out her socks so she got some slippers at Walmart. Her daughter nagged her about it when they were at the store together: *Mom, why are you walking like that and c'mon can't you move a bit faster?* Sam told the kid what she could do with her criticisms . . .

The stairs at the entryway to her apartment building were an issue. With her heavy legs Samantha increasingly had to use the railings to pull herself up and she held on tight for balance on the way down too. One day she slipped on a stair going down, her feet went sideways out from under her and she came down hard, *Thwack!* on her rump before bouncing her head off the base of the adjacent wall. She saw stars but didn't pass out. An odd burning tingle started in her feet and pinkie fingers, so she sat for a while hoping it would all go away. But it didn't. Eventually she hauled herself up, wobbled into her place and managed to get dinner ready.

The tingles didn't go away. The shuffle didn't go away. Samantha could live with all that, at first.

By first snow, the tingling in her hands was bugging her a lot. It was there all day every day and even woke her up at night. She was having trouble holding stuff like knives and forks. Doc said it might be a pinched nerve in her wrist so she had some nerve testing done and that confirmed carpal tunnel syndrome. Knowing that, Sam decided that she could live with the symptoms. No, she didn't want that surgery on the nerves to her hands.

In November, she started tripping in the house, just in the morning at first but more and more every day so she was back to the doctor about it. After another brief examination of her hands and feet the doctor said she would refer Samantha to see a neurologist, a nerve specialist.

The neurologist was a nice, very serious, young fellow who spent a long time talking to Sam about all her troubles and who examined her, not just her hands and feet but he asked her to stand and walk and do all kinds of gymnastics too. He said he was worried because she wobbled so much. There could be a spinal cord problem and she should have an MRI done. Soon.

Why soon? The neurologist explained that if there were bone spurs or disc bulges or something damaging Samantha's spinal cord, the cord might scar and then she'd never be normal again. She'd been symptomatic and getting worse for over a year as it was, and the worse you are coming into it, the less the odds of improvement with surgery.

The family doctor called her back the day after her scan, all upset. Yes, there was a disc bulge compressing Sam's spinal cord in a big way. In fact there were several. The report said some were in her neck and some were lower down between her shoulder blades. No way for the doctor to know which was most important, but she did know that a patient like Samantha needed to see a surgeon pronto and so she'd already made an appointment for Sam later that week.

Could Sam see the scan? No, the scan's at the hospital and we're at the office. The doctor didn't see the actual scan or know how to read it. She just read the report and told Sam they had to trust the radiologist.

The surgeon was a nice guy, polite and caring. Didn't spend a lot of time interviewing or examining Samantha because he had the neurologist's note, which was apparently "quite thorough." He started off with looking at her hands, concerned that the muscles were visibly shriveling and her fingers starting to bend. He talked about myelopathy hand being a bad thing. He tested her arm and leg reflexes with his hammer and watched her walk a bit. Then he left her sitting alone in his examining room forever while he looked at the scan.

When he came back he talked a lot and fast, said he saw six different bulges and spurrings in the front of her neck behind her throat and they all looked bad, and there were even more lower down through the length of her spine. He couldn't remove them all because it would be massive surgery and almost certainly kill her, if not both of them. Apparently the best thing to do for a case like this was not to remove all the bulges at all but to leave them there and do a big laminectomy operation on the back of the spine to open the nerve channel and make more room for the spinal cord. If the disc bulges had made the space smaller, let's make the space bigger! That made sense to Sam.

The surgeon said that the higher up towards the brain on the spinal cord a bulge was, the more important it became, so operating on the discs in her neck was the first priority. Also, opening the spinal canal with a laminectomy weakened it and so he'd have to put a bunch of screws and rods in there to strengthen things too — yes, all at the same time, just one operation. That would stiffen her neck but there was just no way around it. Made sense. Was this a big operation, Doc? Would she need transfusions? Mom got liver poisoning from a transfusion and Samantha would rather die than have any serious complications. Yes, this was not a small operation but not a huge one either. She might bleed enough to need transfusion but that didn't usually happen. *Her life, her risk,* Doc said. The surgeon also explained that her spine had her on the way to a wheelchair, so Sam really was between a rock and a hard place. Samantha signed two different forms, one accepting surgery and another refusing transfusion under any circumstances. Or at least she tried too. Her hands and fingers were so numb and spastic that she could barely hold the surgeon's expensive-looking pen.

Waking up from surgery was not fun. The back of Sam's neck was a mass of pain, her vision was blurry and she was nauseated and barfy. At first her arms and legs didn't feel any different at all.

She couldn't sleep that first night because she was in too much pain and nurses bugged her around the clock with *What's your pain on a 10-point scale?* every hour on the hour.

By morning the pain was settling, but she was so drugged up she was loopy and slurring her words a bit when the surgeon came by to see her, so much so that he assessed her for stroke after examining her arms and legs. No stroke. He explained that the surgery had gone well in terms of opening her spinal canal and that he'd seen her spinal cord swell up to a normal diameter as he did the work. There'd been a small problem though. The thin membrane called the *dural sac*, which contains the spinal fluid surrounding the spinal cord, had torn a bit and she'd lost some spinal fluid as it leaked out. That was why she'd been so barfy and it explained her blurry vison too. He'd sewn up the tear and stopped the leak so she'd feel better soon. Let's hope so . . .

A week later the pain was down to a dull roar and Sam could think straight. She was still barfy, but her hands felt better, less numb and a bit stronger and better able to hold the pen when she filled out her menu forms. Her legs didn't feel any better though; if anything they felt weaker. She was having trouble lifting them to boost herself up onto the bedpan so the nurses brought out this big power lifter thing to hoist her onto it. That helped. But when they used it to try getting her out of bed and into a chair, she developed a huge headache and a rush of nausea after just a few minutes so she hit the buzzer and they put her right back to bed.

Next day, same thing again.

The sixth day after surgery Sam woke up with her pillow all wet. The nurse thought Sam was leaking spinal fluid and immediately called the surgeon. He ordered the nurse to keep Samantha NPO, which meant she couldn't eat or drink, while an emergency MRI was arranged.

Shortly after the scan her surgeon explained that yes, there was an ongoing spinal fluid leak in her neck. He apologized for it and thought maybe his stiches from the repair had torn out. He said the best thing to do would be to return Sam to the operating room to repair the leak, and he started to blah blah blah about using patches and BioGlue and all sorts of technical stuff. *Where do I sign, Doc?* Surgery happened a few hours later.

Next morning Samantha finally felt much better, no headache at all and completely clear-headed. Her surgeon came by wearing a worried expression but when she answered his question about how she felt, he broke out into a great big grin and high-fived the nurse. He told her the repair had gone "Great!" and she'd be fine now, though because of her still-weak legs she'd need extensive inpatient rehab and he'd be putting her on a transfer list for that.

A month later she was still hospitalized in rehab and struggling to walk even with the support of parallel bars. Really her legs weren't getting stronger at all. Not much pain, just very weak. The rehab doctors weren't happy, and when one morning her left hand was a bit more wonky than it had been the day before, they said she should have another scan "just in case." Off to radiology a third time.

Next day another surgeon came by to see Sam, explaining that her doctor was away and he was on call for the day. The scan had shown a big fluid density in her neck, deep enough inside that nothing was leaking out but big enough to be compressing her spinal cord almost as badly as it had been originally. Nobody could be 100 percent sure what it was. According to radiology, infections and blood clots could look like this, but the surgeon said he thought it was almost certainly spinal fluid. Whatever it was, because the spinal cord was compressed and her hand rapidly losing strength, she should be off to the OR a third time for it to be drained out. *OK, where do I sign?*

Not so fast this time. This surgeon asked her about her legs a great deal, concerned that she had not gained any strength there. Samantha explained that never mind not gaining, she had *lost* strength since she'd been in hospital. Surgeon 2 examined her legs and feet again, tested her strength and ability to feel and did a really odd thing with her big toes, wiggling them up and down and asking her to tell him what was up or down — she couldn't tell, which was really weird.

He launched into a long-winded talk about how her spinal cord had been squished at so many places throughout her neck (cervical spine), chest (thoracic spine) and low back (lumbar spine). The new scan confirmed that the laminectomy operation had widened her spinal canal enough to relieve pressure on the cord from the discs in front of it, but there were several equally severe compressions in the upper chest below the neck, and then one more way down in the low back area. Her first surgeon had done the right thing for her hands, obviously, but with her legs getting worse there was clearly more decompressing to be done. Where to do it?

Surgeon 2 explained that, as in the neck, compressions in the chest can affect either the spinal cord or the nerve roots, or both sometimes. However, the spinal cord ends at the top of the low back, so the lumbar spine actually has no spinal cord in it — only a bunch of nerve roots. Compressions of those nerve roots dull your hammer-tap reflexes at the ankle and knee, whereas spinal cord compressions in the cervical or thoracic spine have the opposite effect, increasing them.

Sam's knee and ankle reflexes were so jumpy that the problem compression had to be higher up than the low back, in her chest. The compression in her low back apparently wasn't all that bad and would certainly not explain an inability to stand up or lift a leg off the bed. So, this surgeon said if Sam was going back into the OR to have the spinal fluid leak repaired, he'd want to decompress between her shoulder blades to help her spinal cord at that level while he was in there. It would be a relatively small add to what would be her third operation now, with a lot of potential upside.

Makes sense. When Sam signed up, her signature was already much better than it had been. And again she asked to sign the "no transfusions" form.

Whoops. She'd already had two operations fairly close together in time and so Surgeon 2 checked her blood counts. Her hemoglobin was in the low 80s; normal for a woman is around 110–130 and the heart starts to be starved of oxygen around 65. So that was a concern. He explained in very straightforward terms, a bit rude really, that if bleeding became a problem, there was very real potential now for her to die. *Go ahead Doc, I can't live like this.*

Off to the OR. Reopen the wound, let out the puddle of spinal fluid, sew up the ongoing spinal fluid leak with one teeny tiny 6-0 Prolene suture that's thinner than a human hair, just one stitch in the right place is all it took.

And let's not forget five more laminectomies between the shoulder blades. There was a time that was a Great Big Thing, but not so much in capable hands today. This surgery is tough to do compared to the neck because the flesh is deep and strong, so hard to work through, and the upper thoracic laminas are thick and hard to cut away. Samantha didn't need stabilizing implants this time because the strong short upper ribs give a lot of strength to the spine.

Waking from this operation was easier. Sure, Sam was sore from the bigger cut, but there was no nausea and no vomiting. She actually felt pretty good. Her legs didn't ache at all, and the left side was much stronger even in the recovery room. She worried about the other side. Doc said give it a chance. Next morning the right leg was a bit stronger too.

Samantha had a smooth recovery from there, slow progressive improvements in strength, dexterity and mobility for a year, helped along the way by several months of inpatient rehab up front and twice that much outpatient work after. Her pain faded entirely and she didn't need any meds. Her balance didn't fully recover, so she'll always need that walker outside the house — in her late 30s. Not a great life but better than a wheelchair and she's able to live at home with family to help her.

SPINE CRIMES

This is a tough one for me. There are enough spine crimes here that if they were all attributed to one individual, it might warrant capital punishment! But the case does really illustrate the problem with a profound ignorance of red flags, the critical indicators of spine pathology. This is a big enough issue not only among the general public but especially within the medical community. Let's summarize the glaring red flags we find here in Samantha's case:

1. You'd think a person would speak out about feeling so weak and numb and tingly that they're falling down and can barely use their hands. You'd think a person would demand help from their doctor or the emergency room. But the under-privileged in our society often have little voice, and when they do present to health care, we medicals often dismiss them because if they don't have back pain, it can't be a spinal problem, right? When "they're not like us," we often don't ask people the right questions or take the time to do a proper examination.

2. When Samantha first complained about her cold feet, the doctor might have asked about her ability to stand and walk and the shuffling problem might have prompted some workup, or at least brought the doctor to ask her patient to stand and walk a bit in the office. At that point Samantha might already have had neurological gait abnormalities, which are easy to miss at the bedside examination. She might have been a bit spastic by that point too. Her issues could have been detected and treated earlier had there been even simple diagnostic testing and observation.

3. Ditto on that first neurologist doing the EMG. Obviously the reason for the test — "numb tingly hands" — was not pursued one iota. If the doctor had asked a few probing questions, Sam would have described numbness in *all* of her fingers; median nerve compression at the wrist or carpal tunnel syndrome doesn't do that. A few simple questions might have picked up the shuffling/stumbling complaint and trouble with power and fine motor control in the hands — carpal tunnel syndrome doesn't usually do that either. We shouldn't be surprised that the EMG test was positive because minor carpal tunnel compression and corresponding symptoms are very common in people who work regularly with their hands in any way. Tests and imaging should only be relied on to support a diagnosis and help us determine how best to treat the problem if needed. But the test doesn't *make* the diagnosis, the *symptom history* does, and we must take the time to elicit it.

4. Spinal fluid leak is always a risk of spine surgery. In my training, it was taught as a 1 to 2 percent event, but modern literature quotes rates up to around 10 percent. They can be hard to fix, and it doesn't always go right the first time. That was no crime, but picking your decompression, doing the easy bits and leaving serious residual pressure on the patient's spinal cord, is a spine crime that is committed way too often.

5. Surgeon 1 wrote a full decompression off as "too much surgery," and Samantha was very lucky to have the ongoing issue recognized by Surgeon 2 in a timely way, and to make the recovery she did, albeit partial. I'd say the most common surgical error that brings patients back is under-operating, not doing enough to fix the whole problem. If this patient had come to Surgeon 1 with weak rubbery legs, a normal neck MRI and thoracic compression — which Samantha also had — he'd have operated in a heartbeat. It's inexcusable that he stopped treating his patient after doing the neck.

Sam got really lucky that her rehab doctor cared enough to rescan her persisting weakness rather than simply writing her off with "there was too much spinal cord damage for a good recovery." The delay ruined her life. Surgeon 1 got in there quickly enough to get her hands back to virtually normal, but another several weeks of critical spinal cord compression left her on a walker in her 30s.

Yes, big surgery takes its toll on both the patient and the surgeon, but when it's too much for one go, there are workarounds. One might ask a colleague to step in and do the second half after we do the first. Or split up the surgery by a few days or a week; do two smaller operations rather than one monster. Surgeon 1 never seems to have thought of any of that. His patient suffers for it every day.

Chapter 8

Herman the Hip Arthritis Patient

Nerve pain is not always obvious.
Neither is the risk of doing the wrong
operation!

A t 80 Herman was who we all hope to be in our golden years: a busy, active and independent senior easily able to live on his own, travel a bit, do volunteer work and remain active in the community. He was all the kids' favorite great-grandpa!

His hip had been sore for a long time but he could put up with it, and you don't get to be an independent octogenarian by running off to the doctor with every little ache and pain. But when the limp started, that got him thinking, and as the limp worsened he made up his mind to get it checked out.

At the clinic, a nice young man around his grandson's age took his medical history and after examining him asked about his pain and what treatments he had had for it. None? Why not? Let's start.

Over the next few months and through several visits to the clinic, Herman tried Tylenol and an anti-inflammatory and then a few different non-narcotic pain relievers, all the while going to physio where he felt he was wasting his time as somebody massaged his hip and stretched his legs a bit. He got a better stretch on his morning walk, limp or no! The physios reported a lot of spasm in his back and hip muscles so the doctor prescribed an anti-spasm medication that made Herman feel loopy. He returned it to the pharmacy after two days. Finally the doctor ordered some X-rays and the report came back with a diagnosis: Herman had arthritis in his hip! Would he consider seeing a surgeon?

No, it's not that bad.

FIRST CONSULT

Six months later it was, and Herman met a neat middle-aged woman with silvering hair who listened to his story and examined him. When she poked around his groin and thigh he was a bit tender there for some reason. After looking at the X-rays she showed them to Herman, pointing out how his right hip joint was very perfectly round and the left was flattened a little bit, the cartilage space gap between the bones was thinner and there was a small spur just above the hip on the bone of the pelvis. Apparently the arthritis here wasn't terrible, but this doctor explained that treatment decisions are best made in tune with the patient's symptoms and disability. Sometimes a terribly arthritic hip isn't very painful and so nothing needs to be done, but when there is a lot of pain or disability, it is time. By this point Herman's leg was rubbery and he'd stumbled a few times, so it was time to do something.

But was surgery at his age a smart thing? Herm learned that hip replacements at his age are quite common. They are usually done with a spinal (epidural) anesthetic where he'd be awake but frozen from the waist down, rather like for childbirth, and there was an exciting newer anterior surgical approach which could be done through a small cut in the groin that didn't hurt much. He'd be out of the hospital the next day, sore from the incision for a month or so and would take off like a rocket after that. Didn't sound so bad, and Herman was willing to sign up, but first the surgeon had a concern. Yes, you're over 80 years old so let's avoid surgery if you can. She wanted him to have an X-ray-guided injection of freezing and cortisone into his hip to see if that would help. He did, and it didn't. So Herman signed up.

FIRST SURGERY

Surgery was interesting. Herman could follow the surgeon's conversation and directions to the assistants as she worked. When the power saw started up the anesthesiologist gave him a short-acting sedative and he dozed off for a bit. Before he knew it, he was in the recovery room talking to the guy in the next bed who'd just had his gallbladder out.

Herm wasn't so happy next morning. There was a great burning pain in his groin and his hip still hurt too. The nurses ran around with pain meds all morning and by noon when the surgeon came by he was settling down but hadn't been up yet. Physio came by with a walker later that afternoon and he lurched around the room a bit.

He was slow getting over it all but by the morning of the fourth day, he was fairly comfortable on his meds and moving well enough to go home. Home care delivered a high toilet seat and a walker to the house, and after that a physiotherapist came in several times a week to help him walk and teach him some strengthening exercises.

A month later he was over the surgical pain and off his meds; the cut and his groin didn't hurt much at all. But his hip still hurt. The surgeon ordered X-rays, pronounced them "A-OK" and sent Herman to the outpatient physiotherapy clinic. Apparently some strengthening would help a lot.

Six weeks later he didn't feel much different and the surgeon was concerned. X-rays were fine again. A worry was that there might be some low-grade infection brewing in the hip and so several blood tests and a nuclear scan were ordered. He was even sent to an allergist to see if he might be the rare patient who was allergic to the metal in the new hip joint. The tests were all negative.

Another six months later the bottom line was that Herman wasn't much different than he had been at square one. The surgeon had a long chat with him, telling him that because the test results were all normal she couldn't prove what was hurting him. She explained that some people got pain from the stresses that these implants put on the bone around them and she volunteered to revise the operation, to take out what was in there and try Herman with another type of hip replacement that might be better tolerated.

No dice, Doc, if it didn't work once why should it work a second time? Thank you for trying, and goodbye.

Six months after that Herman had another chat, this time with his family doctor. Maybe his hip replacement was perfect on his X-rays but his hip hurt, he limped, his leg was rubbery. Any ideas? The doctor ran through his notes, and the physio reports describing spasm in the back muscles caught his eye. He looked further and sure enough all the hip X-ray reports mentioned some disc degeneration in the lower spine just above the pelvis, so maybe there was a *back* problem.

Herman had his doubts because his back didn't hurt but he humored the doctor and had back X-rays done that confirmed a lot of arthritis there, and then he agreed to an MRI. The MRI report was three pages long and the doctor said he wasn't sure what it all meant but it did say Herman had something called *spinal stenosis*, which could be bad and so Herman really should see a spine surgeon.

When Herman asked, "What the hell is a spine surgeon?" his family doctor explained that orthopedic surgeons and neurosurgeons are all licensed to do spine surgery but they don't all specialize in it. A spine surgeon is an orthopod or neurosurgeon who does.

SECOND CONSULT

The spine surgeon was a nice enough fellow. He took a medical history again and after examining Herman had him get up and walk around the office a bit, both with and without his cane. He said that Herm's gait was odd. Hip patients usually lurch sideways, but Herman was whipping his whole bad-side leg forward as if *all* the leg muscles were weak, not just the hip muscles.

Then he did an odd thing; he asked Herman to take a finger and point to where his hip hurt. *Idiot, shouldn't that be obvious?* No, please, show me exactly where the pain is.

Herman scowled and straightened out his gnarly knuckled middle finger and pointed. To the edge of the pelvic bone just above his thigh.

The surgeon grinned. Bingo! That's not your hip; that's nerve pain . . . like sciatica but in the lesser of the two major nerves to the leg, the femoral nerve.

That's crap. Herman schooled the kid. *Sciatica goes to your leg and your foot, lots of my friends have it.*

The surgeon explained that there are two major nerves that supply the leg: the femoral and sciatic nerves. The bigger sciatic nerve is formed mostly from the *lower* nerve roots in the back and travels through the pelvis to exit deep beneath the gluteus muscle of the rump before running down the back of the thigh. The smaller femoral nerve is formed more from the middle and upper lumbar nerve roots and supplies the front of the thigh and the knee. When this nerve is inflamed it can become tender, and that tenderness tends to focus where the nerve escapes the protection of the bony pelvis. The sciatic nerve does that underneath the buttock, the femoral nerve in the front of the leg, at the top of the thigh. Herman could understand that.

The surgeon further explained that Herman's spine was very worn out; every single joint in there was "shot," quite common in seniors. Badly worn-out discs in seniors often don't hurt much, likely because there's not nearly as much motion through the joints between them as there is in a hip or a knee. But the MRI scan showed that in Herman's case, arthritic spurrings opposite two discs were pinching the nerves, oddly not the lower discs where sciatica usually originates but high up at the middle and top of the low back, where the femoral nerve originates.

Sciatic pain is literally a pain in the ass; *sciatica* is a symptom complex that originates there and affects the back of the thigh and lower leg. Thigh and groin pains coming from the spine, that's *femoral neuritis*.

Herman had been a bit tender there even before the hip replacement. Hmm.

He learned that spine surgery to trim out a bone spur or two was a small thing, commonly a day surgery. It worked very well nine times out of 10 (just like hip replacements . . .) when done for the right problem, like Herman's. But given his age Herman should probably be observed in hospital overnight afterwards if he wanted to go ahead with it.

I'll try anything, Doc. Can't play with the great-grandkids no more.

First the surgeon explained that for this surgery Herman would have to go to sleep and be positioned on his tummy. All that could put quite a strain on his heart and lungs, so the surgeon wanted Herman to see a cardiologist and get some heart testing done first. If Herman had an intraoperative cardiac event while lying on his belly, the team couldn't quickly reposition him to pump the chest or spark him with a defibrillator and so . . . OK.

More delays. Herman saw a cardiologist, had an echogram and a nukes (nuclear) test, neither of which revealed great results. The angiogram showed a blood vessel to his heart was in fact blocked, a very important one called the *LAD* and so the cardiologist ballooned it and put a stent in there, something like a small piece of mesh tubing to keep the blood vessel open. These stents could develop clots and so Herman would have to take blood thinners for six months before they could safely be interrupted for the surgery. Another delay.

SECOND SURGERY

This was excellent. Herman woke up nauseated and almost threw up before the nurses could get some Gravol into him. His back hurt, a bit. But his original pain was gone.

He went home the next morning as planned and was sore from the cut for about three weeks again. His leg felt stronger under him even as he was leaving the hospital, not perfect but certainly a bit stronger right off.

When the stitches came out a few weeks later Herman asked about physio but the doctor said he should save his money. Research said self-directed exercise was just as good, and if Herman would take a good long walk every day, that would likely help him build his strength just fine. Of course, he'd always done that!

Two months later Herm couldn't be bothered going to his scheduled follow-up appointment with the surgeon, so he canceled. He felt fine. Now 83 years old, but fine.

SPINE CRIMES

This crazy story is very real. Several times a year I operate on somebody who's had a knee replacement for the sin of having some common middle-aged arthritis in their knee X-rays, when their pain is actually coming from L4 nerve root compression in the spine. Once I operated on three people in one month who had had ineffective hip replacements — ineffective because the real problem was upper lumbar spinal stenosis, like Herman.

There were several spine crimes here:

1. **Crime 1:** both the family doctor and the hip surgeon accepted the complaint of "hip pain" for what it was without pursuing it. Otherwise the family doctor was fine. He made sure a thorough regimen of nonoperative care was ineffective before suggesting a surgical opinion. That's really important. Sometimes even people who are quite badly off and have terrible imaging results will have their pain settle down with the simplest of treatments. I keep way more people away

from the operating room with that same good common sense than I put on the wait list.

2. By most standards, the hip surgeon was OK too. She recognized that symptoms were disproportionate to the imaging and her elderly patient was at high risk in any surgery so she pulled out the last stop and sent him for a hip injection before operating. That's good care. What she didn't do (**Crime 2**) was remember that injecting the arthritic hip with anesthetic freezing should have taken *any* pain originating in the hip away for even just a few hours, just as dental anesthetic takes all toothache pain and feeling away from your sore jaw. When it didn't, that fact should have prompted her to think that her patient's pain might be coming from somewhere else.

3. Painful hip replacements are most commonly infected, loose or just plain worn out. Rarely, patients can be allergic to the metal. When her patient had pain soon after hip replacement, she very appropriately worked him up for infection and allergy. What she failed to do (**Crime 3**) was question her patient closely about the pain. If this was a new *different* pain, compared to what her patient suffered pre-op, it might be a problem at the surgical site, but when the same old "baseline" problem pain was still there and unchanged despite the anatomy of the hip having been dramatically altered (removed, really) by surgery, good basic common sense should have prompted the thought that the pain might be coming from somewhere else.

4. One other terrifically common mistake (**Crime 4**) was narrowly avoided by having the patient see a cardiologist beforehand. Surgery in the elderly generally brings much more risk and more complications than does treating healthy younger people, so many surgeons do all they can to avoid it. Hospitals and insurers don't usually record your successes in

care, but they do report complications, which are costly to deal with and the surgeon who has a lot of them is often out of a job.

To their credit, neither the hip surgeon nor the spine surgeon hesitated to treat this very senior patient one iota. The hip surgeon appropriately arranged the safer spinal anesthetic and used a special anterior surgical approach that's a huge technical fiddle but likely better for the patient.

The spine surgeon knew enough and cared enough to think proactively about his patient's cardiac risk. Older spine patients often have a lot of "silent" cardiovascular disease. They might have the worst angina in the world without knowing it because they can't be active enough to stress their hearts (because of the stenosis, remember)! Research has suggested that about 15 percent of spinal stenosis patients' hearts are badly enough off to warrant stenting before the spine surgery, or sometimes even more aggressive procedures.

So, in just one case again we find four spine crimes. Notice that none of them goes to advanced technical issues in care or relates to failed surgery. Nowhere here was the laser offline or the scanner lined up wrong or the robot on the fritz. The surgical microscope was fine and the minimally invasive equipment performed perfectly. These were all failures of basic clinical medicine, not failures of caring or performance but failures to back up our evidence-based knowledge of treatment guidelines with a healthy (and maybe a gently skeptical?) dose of good common sense.

Good doctoring isn't a hard thing, but common sense isn't on any medical school curriculum anywhere that I've ever heard of. Maybe that's another crime.

It's a great pleasure to give our adult patients back to their families so much better off. But we don't expect to meet their kids, grandkids or great-grandchildren at the office . . .

Chapter 9
Brian the Teenager Skipping School

Spine surgery's not for kids, right?

G reat big strapping 16-year-old boys have a shot at a lot of summer jobs that most of their buddies just can't do. Five foot nine and 176 pounds of muscle, Brian could do a lot of manual labor that even many grown men couldn't. The best pay he could find was on a local loading dock doing summer holiday replacement, and it worked out so well that the next summer he was back, two inches taller and eleven pounds heavier.

One day towards end of shift, Brian slipped over the edge of the dock to land on his rear with a *Whump!* on the hard concrete deck below. He winded himself and fell over panting for a few minutes, trying to get his breath back as his coworkers rushed to him.

This overgrown man-child with a beard was crying. His back *hurt*. He stayed on his side curled into a little ball, and when the crew tried to straighten him out, pain just shot through him. So, an ambulance was called at the same time that his buddies called his parents and everybody came together at the ER.

ERs don't generally see a lot of children's injuries and everybody worries about a kid even when they're big and hairy, so Brian got a lot of attention fast. The senior ER doc came to his side, took the story and examined him, wearing a worried expression that scared Brian and got his mom crying. Brian was pronounced "neurologically intact," but because he was in so much pain, X-rays were called for.

First problem: to do spine X-rays in the ER you have to lie on your back and Brian hurt too much. So he was back to the ER and after his parents signed a consent form, the nurses started dripping pain medicine into his IV. An hour later his pain was eased enough to get those X-rays done. They were normal.

But the doctor wasn't happy because Brian had so much pain. Common sprains and strains weren't like this. He worried Brian might have a disc hernia and wanted a CT scan done. Even most disc injuries didn't hurt this much in the ER doctor's experience, and if this was a disc, it would likely have to come out or else paralysis might set in. Dad signed another consent. The CT scan was normal too.

By this time, Brian had had enough IV fluid poured into him that he had to pee. When a nurse brought him a urinal he was horrified and too embarrassed to even try. After the nurse explained what a catheter was he forced himself to stumble off to a bathroom and after that a discussion ensued between Brian, his parents and the doctor. It was agreed he go home with prescriptions for pain medicine and a plan to see the family doctor in a few days.

A few days later he still needed the pills just to get up and move around the house. Getting to the doctor's office in Dad's car was hell. His GP examined him and for a second time Brian heard he was "neurologically normal."

Normal my eye, Doc, there's nothing normal about this.

The doctor thought physiotherapy would help and asked Brian to come back in two weeks, explaining he'd likely be better by then and able to get back to work for a few weeks before school started. He wasn't. More meds, more physio.

Brian's pain didn't settle. At all. It was awful. He could almost control it by hobbling around halfway bent over, but any movement from that position killed. He couldn't sit, he could only lie in the fetal position in bed and Mom or Dad had to help him shower because he couldn't straighten out enough to reach the shower head.

A month of physiotherapy didn't help at all. Then a chiropractor, an osteopath and even a massage therapist. Nothing helped.

Summer was over and now Brian was missing school. He was quickly falling behind so Mom took to homeschooling him. That didn't go well either. It's hard to do well at your lessons lying on your side and halfway seeing double from all those meds.

At a visit just before Christmas, the family doctor had a "frank talk" with Brian and his parents. He said he thought Brian might just be acting out.

What, he thinks I'm nuts? Some doctor.

He explained to Brian's parents that children (Who's a child?) with disabling back pain complaints commonly act out for "secondary gains." It's a way to get out of school if a kid isn't doing well or maybe being bullied. Brian needed to see a psychologist, and an appointment was made.

Back home Brian argued against it. He'd been top of his class academically, and a foot taller than everybody else, he'd put more than one little twerp in his place for picking on other kids. But Mom and Dad were almost crying with worry so he decided to suck it up and go.

Waste of time. Lots and lots of time talking quietly with a weird old guy and hours filling out a bunch of online tickbox questionnaires to get a normal neuropsychological diagnosis.

DIAGNOSIS AND CARE OPTIONS

Early in the New Year the GP ordered an MRI scan and the report said Brian had a black disc. He didn't know what that was so maybe Brian should see a specialist. He made appointments with a physiatrist, a neurologist and the pain clinic. Reluctantly, and only when

Brian's parents asked about it, he referred to a spine surgeon too. The family doctor knew that spine surgery didn't work for back pain, and it wasn't for teenagers.

The physiatrist talked a lot about exercise and behavior and pain and wanted Brian to go back to another physiotherapist who was "very professional." *Pfft!*

The neurologist said the black disc was a "common degenerative abnormality" and didn't mean anything as long as there was no bulge or neurological compression (pinched nerves). He couldn't help.

At the pain clinic they said they could freeze him with a cortisone injection and he'd be fine. Insurance would cover it. That didn't work either.

The spine surgeon took Brian's medical history and examined him like everybody else had. Then she asked Brian to stand up and walk around and try to touch his toes. Brian's fingertips could almost reach his kneecaps. But when he tried to straighten up, he had to arch his spine backwards with his butt sticking out, then grab at his thighs for a second to support himself before straightening out.

Hmm. Let's get some more X-rays done standing up. Brian hobbled off.

When he came back, the surgeon showed Brian and his parents the images from the MRI that had been done earlier, explaining the elementary anatomy and pointing out how one disc, second from the bottom, was black whereas the rest were a light gray color, almost white. She also pointed out how the bone marrow next to that black disc was discoloured a bit (called *Modic changes*), which suggested the black disc was inflamed. She explained that discs are built something like a squishy jelly donut that has no hole and blackening meant the jelly had dried out — a common thing seen in aging discs. (*I'm 17!*) In the MRI, when Brian was relaxed and lying down on his back, his spine didn't look too bad. But then the surgeon brought up the new X-rays and even Brian could see that the shape of his spine in the standing position was very different.

As soon as Brian stood up for his X-rays, everything collapsed; seen from the side, it looked like everything was pitched forward and that one disc (L4/L5) was squished thin a bit in the back and almost completely in the front. You could just about see the bones touching together there. The "hydraulic support" function of Brian's disc had been lost. Surgery could fix that in one of two ways: Brian could have a disc replacement or a fusion.

Brian learned that artificial disc implants were a thing, first approved for use in North America in 2004. Research said they were as good as the old-fashioned fusion operations when used in the right patient who was ideally young, had only one bad disc and no facet arthritis in the bony joints behind the disc. In the X-rays and MRI, Brian's facets looked OK but this surgeon would want him to have a facet block test done first to prove that those joints were not already painfully damaged. If they were, he'd likely stay sore after a replacement.

She explained that artificial discs are inserted with an anterior-approach operation, working through the patient's belly. *Sheesh!* There are at least two major complications to worry about with that. One is that the big blood vessels flowing to and from the legs are plastered atop the spine at L4/L5, and the surgeons would have to mobilize (move) them to get to Brian's Modic disc underneath. Also, the nerves to Brian's "naughty bits" were right there too and they could be damaged at the surgery — Brian's sex life might be over before it had really started!

Nope! Not for me. Just do the fusion through my back.

The surgeon cautioned that, historically, back-dominant pain patients like Brian who had a disc fused did well only about 70 percent of the time. That didn't mean that 70 percent of Brian's pain would go away. It meant that if the surgeon operated on 10 cases like Brian, three people might come out of it absolutely no better off. The rest would be better — but not usually perfect. Pain scores commonly went from 7 to 8 out of 10 to 3s and 4s. But in Brian's case, because of the instability documented in the standing

X-rays, the surgeon said she'd be very surprised if he didn't get very much better.

None of this sounded great. *Do I have to do anything? What if I do nothing?*

No, there was no neurological catastrophe looming and if Brian could live with his pain and limited lifestyle so could the surgeon. But with a longstanding mechanical pain problem there was no miracle cure in Brian's future either, and he'd already tried all the reasonable nonsurgical care options. For the foreseeable future nothing much would change and as he got old he might grow some bone spurs, which tend to stabilize an aged or injured spine and relieve pain.

The surgeon returned to the fusion option, explaining that the standing X-rays proved that Brian's spine wasn't just painful but mechanically unstable. The structure of his spine was like a subtly broken leg. Maybe lying down, the bones of that leg would line up normally and X-rays could look OK; but try to stand on it and *Whammo!* that leg would bend and collapse like Brian's L4/L5 disc did. One could easily understand how the broken-leg patient would be better off when a surgeon drilled a rod through the length of the injured bones, and a mechanically unstable spine was very similar.

The surgeon explained that spine fusion caused one or more vertebrae to grow together and function as one, relieving stresses and load on the disc and joints between those bones. For Brian the ideal would be to remove what was left of his L4/L5 disc and then realign and support his spine there with implants and a bone graft fusion done right where the disc used to be. He'd need some screws to support it too. No, the screws didn't have to come out later; they'd stay in there like a pin in his broken leg or screws in his ankle would. This surgery could be done in several different ways: from the back (a posterior approach), through an anterior approach like disc replacements or even with an approach from the side of the body. It could be either open (making a formal cut) or with minimally invasive technique. This surgeon liked to work from the back and make a cut. She said she could see things better and felt the work was safer that way.

Would the cut hurt?

Of course, but it's just a cut: they heal quickly and don't hurt after that. Brian would stay in hospital overnight for observation and so that the recovery room team could make sure his pain was under control before going home the next morning. He would likely need some mild daily narcotics for about three weeks and would be given prescriptions for those. When he was past that pain and the wound was well healed, the surgeon would prescribe some exercises to help him regain his strength. He'd have to take it easy for three or four months until the bone fusion took, then he could do whatever he wanted.

Will my back get stiff?

Brian, you're stiff as a board *now*. And your spine is wobbly, unstable and more mobile than normal! You're stiff because your back muscles are spasming involuntarily all the time to keep things from wiggling in there. If the surgery works and your pain goes, that spasm will relax and you'll end up just about as normal as the next person. No, the L4/L5 level will never move again, but *the rest* of the body around it would move quite normally and the loss wouldn't be enough for most people to notice.

Brian's parents had heard that fusions were a bad thing and that the patient who has one often ends up needing a second and a third and so on. The surgeon explained that this was true of the degenerated spine common in older patients, whose scans usually show wear and tear at many places other than the surgical site. The odds of something else going bad and needing reoperation for those people are known to be about 3 percent per year of life. But Brian wasn't those people, he was the rare case of an isolated disc injury in an otherwise healthy and well-aligned spine and so his future prognosis was likely much better, possibly even normal.

The family discussion was intense. Nobody was sure, so at first no decision was made. They all went back to the trusted family doctor to discuss things, and he was skeptical, suggesting a second surgical opinion would be a good idea.

Brian and his family met another surgeon the next week. After looking at the MRI without really talking to Brian or examining him, he said there was no neurological compression so nothing could be done; Brian would just have to live with it.

INTERVENTION

Brian decided to go for it with Surgeon 1, and she operated in the late spring. The experience went exactly as hoped. Brian woke up sore from the cut but with his old pain gone. By the time his stitches came out he was able to stand straighter and more comfortably than he had in over a year.

By midsummer Brian was quite comfortable so he enrolled in night school to finish the high school curriculum. Having lost two years of schooling, he didn't want to hang with all the younger kids he'd otherwise be stuck beside in class during the day. He was comfortable sitting for hours, and getting back to studying after so long was easy — he aced it. The next spring he enrolled at the university.

'Nuff said.

SPINE CRIMES

Seventy percent odds of relieving nonspecific back pain with fusion surgery aren't great, and that challenged fact is where spine surgery has acquired a lot of its generally bad reputation. But when a patient is in such severe pain that they're almost completely disabled, and where every other reasonable alternative has been tried and failed, a 70 percent chance at a better life may not be such a bad thing. Abandoning the patient to a life of misery because the odds aren't perfect is a spine crime no matter how old (or young!) the patient is.

Back pain from spinal instability is different from deformity. With lesser degrees of deformity, it's quite common for the spine joints to wear out to the point where one bone will tilt or twist or slide out of perfect alignment with the next. But if things are mechanically stable in that misalignment, the patient's usually fine.

But mechanically unstable patients like Brian are in agony as soon as they stand up. The back muscles spasm and nothing budges in there, and the scientific literature analyses confirm that X-rays and scans done when the patient is lying down commonly don't detect the problem. But they still get done because they're easy and convenient and traditional.

Imagine trying to walk around on an ankle or knee that's going sideways out of joint because all the ligaments are torn up. X-rays of that ankle often look great when the weight's off the leg, so an orthopedic surgeon knows to ask for standing or weight-bearing X-rays (also sometimes called *stress views*) to confirm the diagnosis. That's very standard in orthopedic trauma practice today. Nobody tells those ankle patients to suck it up and take narcotics or visit the pain clinic to be "managed" permanently. They're ordered a brace and crutches and commonly sent for reconstructive surgery to repair their damaged ankle ligaments.

A lot of back pain patients do end up being referred to the pain clinic, and many can do well there. Successful spine injections can relieve pain for months and patients are often happy to trade off a few visits every year against a lifetime of narcotics and disability. But I'd say the pain clinic should be a "port of last call," and that chronic pain patients should be sent there only when problems that can be effectively treated surgically have been thoroughly ruled out.

Too often that doesn't happen . . .

Chapter 10
Patricia's Chronic Back Pain

Whose pain "management" masked her
spinal stenosis until it was too late.

M any people would say that life starts to go downhill after 50 as this and that starts to hurt. As we generally start slowing down, weight and blood pressure and blood sugar commonly go up. Sleep is disrupted. We might lose someone we love to the big C or other illnesses and start to consider our own mortality.

Patricia had had a good first half. She'd raised two great girls with Jeff and enjoyed a rewarding career as executive assistant to a senior banker, a fascinating job where she got to meet a lot of interesting and often powerful people. But backache became a part of life in her 50s. A great benefits plan let her see the massage therapist and physio just about whenever she wanted, and they helped a lot. She kept a bottle of Tylenol in her desk, took the odd one at first and then daily before moving on to Advil. Eventually she needed Tylenol No. 1 with some codeine in it, although that made her very constipated. One day her great family doctor suggested she try the local pain clinic where maybe a cortisone shot would help.

Wouldn't that just hurt more? Not likely, it's just a needle stick in your back like the ones you got when the kids were born. *Oh yeah.* Off she went.

At the pain clinic, she met a nurse practitioner who politely took her symptom and treatment history before examining her. He suggested Patricia have an MRI scan before treatment was started because treatable pathology should be ruled out.

Pathology? You think I have cancer? No, no, no, pathology just means something abnormal in general, and we're just being careful.

When the doctor at the pain clinic explained the MRI report, he said it showed that Patricia had "extensive degeneration" at "all levels" in her spine but there was no compression of the nerves or spinal cord so no surgery was indicated. He also said that in her case a trial injection of epidural steroids might help. He couldn't guarantee anything and, at best, odds were 50/50 she would get relief, but if it did help it would likely last several months. The clinic helped many patients who came in two or three or four times a year for their shots, getting good pain relief and staying off the oral meds. It was a small thing to do and quite safe. Why not try, what's to lose?

Nothing to lose. Everything to gain. The procedure room was available so Patricia gowned up, put on some radiation protection equipment and watched on the monitor as the long "spinal" needle was worked into her spine, a bit of white liquid X-ray dye injected to make sure the needle was in the right place, and the cortisone flowed in.

Next morning she did feel a bit better and so she put her usual Tylenol No. 1 in her pocket and went to work without taking it. She felt fine during the day but by nightfall she was sore, so she took that tablet at bedtime.

Next morning she was better again, and *that* night she passed entirely on her Tylenol.

A month later the pain clinic called her and she was doing well so she declined to go back in for another shot. They asked that she call when and if. OK.

Four months later she called. Same experience again.

That went on for over a decade. Patricia had retired at 62 over the protests of her younger boss who said he couldn't live without her. A young new hire took the job, and Patricia spent a year on the phone helping the poor woman to get it all right.

Approaching 70, Patricia's backache was acting up and the injections weren't lasting very long. She was also finding it harder and harder to get to the pain clinic because her backache was starting to affect her standing and walking. When she had to be on her feet for a long time, waiting for the bus and walking through the hospital to get to the clinic, she'd have to pause and rest quite often.

She talked to the pain doctors about it and they said people can get "habituated" to their meds and the benefit wears off. They suggested they try injecting some stronger drugs. Through a half dozen monthly visits different options and combinations of injectable drugs were tried, and nothing worked.

The next step for chronic pain was to try oral or patch-type narcotic medicines. Pills didn't do too much but a patch worked great and Patricia only had to change it every three days. Her pain was gone! She hadn't had relief in years and she was almost tearfully thankful. Her pain doctor was tearful as well when he announced his coming retirement and the need to pass on her care.

Eight months later she needed a stronger patch and the new young doctor was happy to prescribe it. Six months after that she was back at the clinic because she needed a stronger one again but the doctor was delayed on the phone. She had to wait for her new prescription at the reception counter where after a few minutes her pain was so bad she had to lean on the counter for support, and a few minutes after that her legs quietly gave out from under her and she slowly collapsed onto the floor.

The nurses and one of the doctors came running. They laid her out in one of the exam rooms and checked her pulse and blood pressure, which were fine, before giving her some sweet juice to drink to raise her blood sugar. After a bit, her own doctor came by to ask about what had happened.

Patricia told the story of her leg pains and difficulty standing and walking and how it had been getting worse and worse for a long time.

The doctor examined her on the stretcher and found all her leg muscles to be very weak, especially those at her feet and ankles. He was concerned. Likely it was just because she was old and had been inactive for a long time. But maybe she should have an MRI just in case; she might have pinched nerves or a disc hernia or something. Why not?

The new MRI report was a shocker; it described high-grade spinal stenosis throughout Patricia's low back. This was alarming to the young doctor and so he went through Patricia's files looking for previous imaging reports. There was only one, which was well over a decade old now.

The doctor sat her down for a talk, explained what had been found and suggested Patricia should see a surgeon. Her problem was more than just pain and now involved loss of strength. When a person is so weak they can barely stand up and move around, it's serious and more than time to see a surgeon.

The doctor said he was actually quite relieved to see the MRI report; he'd been worried that Patricia might have a cancer because she'd lost so much weight in recent months. The doctor started to ask a few questions about diet and appetite, and the real problem quickly came to light. Patricia couldn't stand in her kitchen long enough to prepare a decent meal and had been living out of cans for almost a year. Yes, Dear Reader, that's a thing. I see it a lot in my practice.

The surgeon wasn't happy, this spine MRI was "a mess" and Patricia's legs were very weak. He said he could get her nerves anatomically unpinched, or decompressed, but he couldn't promise her she'd ever walk normally again because she was so far gone. Her ability to stand and walk would likely improve a bit (although possibly a lot, and maybe not at all), but something really should be done because she was so weak there was likely a wheelchair in her near future without some surgery.

What about my pain? The surgeon explained that operations for pain were quite unpredictable unless the pain was all related to standing and walking, in which case it would likely get somewhat better just as the strength in her legs would. But the kind of always-there resting or baseline pain that had been Patricia's issue all these years very possibly would persist.

So why have the operation, why go through all that risk if my pain won't go away? Because you can barely stand up and walk and you're pretty much starving to death because of it.

Oh, yeah. Patricia said she'd try surgery.

Patricia awoke after the operation in roaring pain — she was crying and shaking with it. The recovery room nurses were very upset. They gave her pills and injections and put stuff in her IV and nothing worked, so after a few hours of that torture they called the doctor.

After some delay, the spine surgeon came by and spoke with Patricia and her nurses. He was very interested in whether this was "the same old pain" as before surgery or might be a new pain, maybe the pain of the cut. The doctor examined her briefly and found good strength in her legs. Then he looked at the post-op orders and immediately started firing off instructions to the nurses for more and bigger doses of pain meds. Within a half hour Patricia's pain score had been cut in half — and the recovery room nurses' eyeballs had all doubled in diameter!

The doctor apologized to Patricia for all this; apparently the post-op orders were for the standard pain meds prescribed in the hospital. But Patricia was not a standard patient. Having been on high-dose narcotics for some time, she was habituated and needed very high doses to get relief — like a drug addict might.

Now Patricia was upset. *I am not a drug addict!*

The doctor explained, No, of course not. Habituation isn't addiction. It is different and much more benign. It's also common and easy to explain, sort of like the effects of drinking. Remember having your first few sips of beer back in high school? Wow, you were buzzed in no time! But a couple of years later, after some practice, you could handle a beer or two easily and with little effect. This happens because the enzyme systems in your liver that break down alcohol respond to exposure by getting better at it. Winston Churchill won World War II while drinking several bottles of alcohol every day and was always in control of himself! The same thing happens with narcotics: when you use them regularly, your liver gets better and better at metabolizing them and so you need more and more drug to get the same level of pain relief.

With adequate pain control, Patricia was helped onto her feet the next morning by the physiotherapy team and did well. Three days later she was good enough on her feet to go home, after her surgeon's team set up some home care support and Meals on Wheels.

A month later she was ordering groceries online, cooking healthy meals and had gained a few pounds. The surgical pain was largely gone and the old pain felt better too, so she decided to be strong and just stop all those narcotics.

Two days later she was sick as a dog and her neighbor called an ambulance for her. An ER workup found nothing wrong but when the ER staff did a meds check they scolded her for not admitting to all her drugs. *No, I stopped all those on the weekend!*

Patricia learned that you can't just stop high-dose narcotics. A habituated person can go into withdrawal, which makes you feel very sick. They have to be reduced gradually. The ER doctor wrote her out a schedule that cut back her meds a bit every week and would see her down to plain Tylenol in about six months.

Patricia followed her instructions to the letter. She lived into her 90s buying a repeat bottle of Tylenol every other month and never went to the pain clinic again.

Patricia spent years on narcotics she likely didn't really need — and was lucky to avoid serious complications from all that. A common spine crime.

In addition, all the years of stronger and stronger pain meds masked not only Patricia's pain but also the root cause of it. Perhaps if she had been in more pain (because she was on fewer, less potent drugs), more investigation into her back pain would have occurred earlier and more could have been done about it sooner. It's possible that all the pain "management" allowed her spinal stenosis to progress far more than it otherwise would have. Another spine crime.

Failing to reassess the patient and repeat the medical history and physical examination whenever there's a need for a change in treatment or medication, for years, is inexcusable. Fortunately, the new young pain clinic doctor knew her stuff.

I wish more did.

Chapter 11
Spine Care Basics for Primary Care Practitioners and Their Patients

The following essentials of spine care remind us of the common "misses" that, unfortunately and sometimes tragically, occur in primary care. In my opinion, this short list of often neglected spine care truths should be understood by *all* physicians and paramedicals who provide spine care (including physiotherapists, chiropractors, osteopaths and the like) to improve their skills in diagnosing, treating and referring patients who are suffering from back pain and spine-related neurological symptoms.

And patients need to be aware of these spine basics too. If you, the patient, can help bridge the knowledge gap in spine care by bringing informed questions and concerns to your physicians and other caregivers, everybody wins. I learn from my patients every day, and there's no reason you can't become a well-informed advocate for improving spine care!

1. **Ask every back pain complainant to point with one finger to where it hurts, and then investigate that area.**
   Don't rely on the patient's oral report of where the pain is; they may say "my back" or "my hip," but you will get

a much more specific indication of where the problem
is if you ask them to *show* you rather than *tell* you
where it hurts.

2. **Know where the hip is and where hip pain presents**
   (the medial groin), and that the pain patient pointing
   to their buttock likely has sciatica. Sciatic pain is quite
   literally a pain in the ass! We should also distinguish
   between sciatic pain (that sore buttock) and sciatica
   (the leg symptoms of numbness, tingling, weakness and
   so on). The sciatic nerve exits the pelvis to run down
   the back of the leg. This pain is commonly mislabeled
   as piriformis syndrome or sacroiliac joint pain; however,
   those things are very rare whereas sciatic pain is
   extremely common.

3. **Ask a few simple questions about how the pain started.**
   If there was no injury to explain it and it's been present
   for more than a few weeks in a patient with *any* cancer
   history, order a spine MRI of the painful area right away.
   Until proven otherwise, you should assume that patient
   has metastatic spine cancer, which is commonly missed
   on X-rays, CT scans and nuclear medicine tests. Early
   diagnosis in spine metastasis can often avoid neurological
   disaster and/or the need for great big surgery.

4. **Touch (palpate) every back pain patient's back muscles.**
   If they cry out and withdraw at a light touch, it's
   likely that nobody can help them definitively because
   their pain has been psychologically "centralized" and
   "catastrophized" (there are scoring systems for all that).
   Surgery can't fix psychology. Having said that, we've
   read here that uncontrolled spine symptoms can bring
   a person to suicide . . . they can also be responsible for
   extreme anxiety, distress, depression and hyper-reactivity!
   If the symptoms are severe and the scans say there's
   treatable pathology, surgery may be worth a shot.

Chronic back pain patients have been shown to have very abnormal psychometric test results, lots of anxiety and depression and whatnot. Patients with abnormal psychological testing generally don't do as well as others. So, simplistically many surgeons today still deny these people care, saying, "Surgery can't treat psychology." But guess what? When surgery relieves the spine symptoms, and we retest the patients' psychology once they're fully recovered, the psychological testing normalizes a great deal! One surgeon I know likes to call himself a spinechiatrist . . . !

If the back pain patient *doesn't* cry out at your touch and the muscles are in spasm, the patient's spine may be unstable or pathologically malaligned, and if the spasm extends below the waist onto the buttocks, they may be collapsing or have imbalanced deformity. So, especially in these cases, get those standing X-rays!

5. **Ask every back pain patient to stand up and walk.** Are their quads (L3 and L4) strong enough that they can get up from a chair normally? Is their balance good, or are they wobbling with myelopathy? Know what sciatic scoliosis and kyphosis are, and the neurology of drop foot, Trendelenburg gait and a quads lag. Ask people to stand up on their toes to detect S1 deficits — then on each leg if they can do it in tandem. The manual motor examination for strength in the legs, where we push with a few pounds of pressure against muscles that can normally exert hundreds of pounds of force, is very insensitive. People can be so weak that they can barely stand but still examine quite normally to manual stress.

6. **Don't be afraid to get X-rays of your spine pain patient.** The internationally accepted "practice wisely" guidelines (there's a website!) suggest that spine X-rays usually don't tell us much, and when your patient has

just sprained their back, they don't. But when spine pain has been there for weeks or months, it's more than time. Order X-rays even earlier if pain is severe, rapidly escalating or not responding to common care measures. Simple X-rays can reveal a lot when a case isn't evolving as expected.

7. **Get those X-rays done with the patient standing up.** Most patients don't hurt when they lie down, and serious conditions like instability or deformity may not be detected without having the patient stand up!

8. **There are two major nerves to the leg; the sciatic is only one of them.** Remember that pelvis/flank pain running from the waistline bone of the pelvis at your side and down the front of the thigh to the knee isn't always hip pain either — that can be L3 or L4 compression in the femoral nerve distribution. I've operated on many people like this who have either been denied spinal decompression surgery "because there's no sciatica" or had knee replacements done that didn't relieve their leg pain one iota.

9. **Remember pinched nerves often don't hurt.** They have no nerve endings in them to generate pain. Only inflamed nerves hurt. So, the patient complaining only of neurological symptoms often has a spine problem, although they may be completely without spine pain. Cervical myelopathy patients complain that their hands are numb and tingly, or that they're losing fine motor control. Lumbar stenosis patients can't stand or walk more than very short distances. And many of them will have no pain at all.

10. **Remember that the most common first neurological symptom of a pinched spinal cord in the neck (cervical myelopathy) is numbness and tingling** in all the fingers of one or both hands (not just the thumb, index finger

and thumb side of the middle finger, which is more likely carpal tunnel syndrome); and with sciatica, it's numbness in the leg or foot. Many if not most neck cases have no neck pain at all, and up to a third of lumbar stenosis patients present with no back or sciatic pain.

11. **Remember that the most common cause of sudden (often painless) new-onset motor impairment in an adult is likely spinal.** When your patient is suddenly unstable or falling down or having trouble walking, unless they're having an obvious stroke, get an urgent MRI of their spine first, second and third — because these crisis spine conditions can do so well with timely surgery. If the patient is very numb and tingly and their hands and arms are affected, scan the neck. If not, scan the low back. Only if the MRI is negative, when you've ruled out severe and treatable structural disease in the spine that can be a relatively "quick fix" with good prognosis, should you refer to physios and neurologists or the pain clinic.

Part 2

When Surgeons Fail Their Patients

Chapter 12

Anne the Widow

*A surgeon's gold mine. When we get it wrong,
we get paid again to try to fix it!*

There's a population of people whose spines are genetically predisposed to wear out early; sometimes they have end-stage disc degeneration in their 30s. Nothing in the scans of these people looks normal: there's always degeneration everywhere. Many have terrible chronic pain and disability. And surgically we can't usually do a darn thing about it. Anne was one of those genetically cursed people. Her pain started in her 20s and escalated after she had her kids.

The trouble is, back pain isn't really a thing, any more than abdominal pain is. Abdominal pain is not a diagnosis; it's a syndrome that can have many different specific causes, like gallbladder disease, appendicitis, kidney stones and so on.

And just as "belly surgery" cannot cure "abdominal pain," "back surgery" cannot alleviate "back pain." In the spine, we can treat only identifiable causes of pain surgically. We can decompress nerves, stabilize instability, correct deformity. That's all we can do. Even if the spine is massively worn out but isn't compressing nerves or bent out of shape or wobbling around, we usually can't relieve pain by operating.

These long-suffering people are frequently referred to pain clinics as their only option, to have their pain managed in a variety of ways. I hate that term, *managed*. We'd never "manage" your painful hip or knee or shoulder or belly or chest — we'd figure out what hurts and correct it to relieve your pain. We'd never say "take these meds" or "get those shots" for the rest of your life to those people, and you the patient would never accept such direction from us. But in spine care it happens all the time.

I'd like to live in a medical world where every "chronic pain" patient is referred to somebody like me to make sure they aren't candidates for pain-relieving surgery before being labeled as chronic (that is, untreatable). One of my great joys in practice is taking a pain clinic patient to the operating room and knocking it out of the park!

Until she was referred to me, Anne was on the typical path of the chronic pain patient: therapy of various sorts started in her 30s, prescriptions started in her 40s, and by her mid-50s, she was a regular pain clinic client. Never without pain, not able to work or travel much and just barely able to look after herself.

THE TIPPING POINT FOR ANNE

As our discs age and dry out, they collapse and we get shorter. We also tend to pitch forward slightly because the collapsing discs are in the front (anterior) part of the spine and the harder bony posterior part can't collapse very easily. That forward bend in turn increases load on what's left of the discs and they can rupture. That happened to Anne in her mid-60s and that was when she met me, the on-call surgeon that day. She had a great big L3/L4 disc hernia causing crippling sciatic pain burning down her right leg, and she couldn't put any weight on it at all.

Fishing out the disc bulge can take less than an hour, and when the problem is sciatica rather than back pain, it works like a charm. It's been routine day surgery for over 30 years.

After I took Anne's disc hernia out she was happy with the sciatic relief but I was worried. Post-op X-rays showed that the little bit of disc she had left there had collapsed further forward, overstraining the spine. That's a hard place to be for a surgeon; we might see the potential for trouble ahead, but when the patient is doing well, it's not easy to convince anybody that more surgery is indicated. I discussed it with her and she declined further care at that point. With her sciatica gone, her back pain was where it had always been and she could live with that, so she returned to the pain clinic for more "management."

A few years later Anne blew out that same disc again (yes, that's a thing — it happens to about 6 to 7 percent of discectomy patients) and collapsed even further. The surgeon on call that day took the new disc hernia out but sadly he did it with a very old-fashioned laminectomy, a technique that removes significant bone tissue from behind the disc and can weaken the spine structure. It's how disc surgery was first done in the 1930s, but since around the 1970s, we've been making it a smaller and smaller operation. Today, laminectomy is only rarely necessary in treating disc hernia. In Anne's case, it left her even more collapsed, deformed and unstable.

Now her back pain was worse. Much worse than it had ever been. Anne couldn't stand up straight. The narcotics dose that had been stable for years went up.

The pain clinic tried to "manage" her through several more years of misery, more and more drugs and injections and you name it. They got nowhere. Eventually in desperation, Anne asked to be referred back to the surgeon she had seen most recently.

He scanned her again, no pinched nerves and so nothing to do, right? That's what spine care still is to too many surgeons today, pinched nerves or nothing. She wouldn't go away and so he referred her to not one but two colleagues, an orthopedic surgeon and a neurosurgeon. These colleagues had more aggressive practice in spine care; they knew how to put screws into the spine and did fusions and they determined that's what she needed. They decided that this was so complex a case they were going to operate together; it was too much for one surgeon to do. Because the spine was collapsed, the plan was to do a big multilevel fusion across the discs above and below, for "mechanical reasons." Yeah sure. The discs above and below were no different than they'd been for decades. They weren't the problem.

So Anne had a three-level fusion operation done, running from L2 to L5. From years of inactivity, her bones were very soft with osteoporosis and the surgeons had to inject bone cement before inserting the screws, which would otherwise be very loose. So now she was rock-solidly screwed together. And bent forward, very deformed, imbalanced. No hope of ever standing up straight. The narcotics dose went up again.

Anne was so crooked she had to lean on a cane or walker to stop herself from falling forward. That long stiff fusion is known to increase stress on the bones and joints around it. Did either of her two board-certified surgeons prescribe any osteoporosis medicine after operating on her, maybe some basic vitamin D? Nope.

Predictably, within a year there was an osteoporosis fracture of the L1 vertebra above her fusion. She was back to one of her surgeons with more pain. The narcotics dose went up again.

Osteoporosis-related spine fractures are very common; data suggest that up to 700,000 happen in North America alone every year. Most don't amount to much — Granny (or Grandpa) is achy and sore for a bit and the bone heals rapidly. It looks a bit squished in your X-rays but generally doesn't bother the patient much. Of those 700,000 fractures, only one in three comes to medical attention and then two out of three heal like gangbusters without surgery, so just roughly one in nine (call it 10 percent of all these fractures) might need attention.

But Anne's fracture was not an isolated osteoporosis fracture. It was a simple little osteoporosis fracture in a badly deformed spine adjacent to a long stiff fusion construct from the previous surgery and right up against the stiffened thoracic spine opposite the rib cage. Sadly, the same surgeons who thought doing a fusion crooked was a great idea didn't recognize the important unique biomechanical issues with this fracture, and so she was told to go home and rest for a few weeks and it would heal like any other osteoporosis fracture.

It didn't. A month later she was back in the ER, unable to stand up because of the pain and regularly losing control of her bladder. ER physicians examined her and referred her to the on-call spine guy. At the bedside examination, her legs were strong, no deficits neurologically. She could empty her bladder. So she was labeled as a "pain person," the narcotics dose went up again, and she was referred back to the pain clinic.

Nobody in the ER ever asked her to stand up and walk. That's an important part of assessing any spine care patient. The pain patient should always be asked to point with a finger to where it hurts, and the trouble-walking people should always be asked to stand up and walk. Too often these simple things don't happen.

WE MEET AGAIN

A few days later she was back, on a day when I was on call. The poor lady couldn't stand up; she'd been pretty much bedridden at home and crawling to the bathroom. Really!

Despite having been off her feet, a new set of X-rays showed Anne's fracture to be worse, much worse. Not only had it crumbled substantially, I could see that there was a dislocation developing through it — her spine was going "out of joint" as her rib cage and upper body were dissociating from her lower half. Something had to be done. But what?

This unstable fracture had to be stabilized, but remember Anne had had her previous fusion done in a badly malaligned position such that she literally could not stand up without support. Here would be a golden opportunity to take advantage of well-she's-going-to-be-in-the-OR-asleep-anyway and get her realigned. That's a relatively common thing today and can involve a number of different surgical techniques up to and including osteotomy procedures, where we literally just about cut the spine in half and reset its alignment. A formal osteotomy (commonly called a *PSO*) usually gives about 30 degrees of correction, and we can tweak it (trapezoidal osteotomy) with implants to get another 10. These are massive operations that can take all day, bleed several pints of blood and have huge complication risks.

Smaller realignments in the range of 10 degrees or so can be done by jacking up the collapsed disc spaces and implanting support devices (and bone graft for fusion) into them, and again we can tweak those with "release osteotomies" to get maybe another five degrees of correction.

These interbody reconstructions (fusions done within the actual disc space, usually with support implants that help realign the spine) are not small operations either. At my hospital a simple one-level reconstruction sees four hours pass between the patient going into the OR and coming out again. One-third of that is anesthesia time but two-thirds is my work. The patient can easily lose a unit of blood, not enough to need transfusion but enough to create some anemia. It's roughly the same "hit" as a common cardiac operation.

A two-level case needs another hour, and so on and so on. Here we might be looking at *six* different levels. In a debilitated lady in her 70s, that's prohibitive. So what to do?

Spinal alignment is known to change with position. We typically gain 10 degrees of lordosis (low back) curvature simply by going from lying down on our back to standing up. We gain another 10 lying prone (on our belly) on a special spine operating table. People with worn-out collapsed spines can sometimes realign significantly with such simple positioning, and aggressive surgeons can capture that with fixation screws using special techniques. My hope was that Anne's old fusion wasn't well-knit and that if I took out her old screws, she'd straighten out enough to make a difference.

When we have to realign somebody, we always want to do it as low down in the spine as we can. Most of our normal lordosis curvature comes in the lower two lumbar discs, so that's where most degenerative malalignment comes from and that's where it's best corrected.

When planning the surgery, I measured Anne's alignment on standing pre-op X-rays and found that she was actually *50 degrees* collapsed from where she should be! Imagine trying to stand and walk bent forward by 50 degrees! Impossible. Correcting her would need not one but two big PSOs and she'd likely bleed to death. So I decided to get what I could with a smaller procedure, either a pair of those lesser interbody realignments or nudging each (hopefully) mobile disc space with new screws and interbody implants after taking out the old ones.

I booked an all-day OR with an ICU bed for her aftercare and off we went. First impression was bad because even having given her a blood-thickening drug called *TXA* that cuts surgical bleeding, just about anything I touched in there was either muscular scar from all the previous surgery or very soft bone, both of which can bleed a great deal. I'd have to get in and out as quickly as possible. That ruled out any interbody fusion work, which is notoriously bloody.

First step was to take out the old screws . . . but they were cemented in! I got lucky, and the upper pair easily came away from the cement. The lower pair wouldn't budge. There would be no tweaking disc spaces open down there. If I was going to get or hold an improved alignment, it would only be starting at L3/L4.

The operation went well, but surgical care is not over when we close the wound. Too often (in my opinion) spine surgeons forget that. There's a lot we can do after the surgery to potentially improve the outcome. When we fix your broken ankle, we don't let you go jumping around on it the next day. You're in a cast or a splint, and we tell you not to walk on it for quite some time. It's months till we discharge most people. In spine care, too often we forget that.

Because Anne was so deformed and osteoporotic, I took several measures to improve the chances of a good outcome:

1. I put her into a supportive spine brace that stopped her bending forward and required her to wear it for six months. (It generally takes about four months for weight-bearing bone to heal well even in a healthy young person with strong hard bone.)
2. Right after surgery, I gave her an IV bone-hardening drug called *pamidronate*, which is used in hospitals to strengthen bones weakened by cancer metastasis.
3. I started her on vitamin D right away. It stimulates bone cell metabolism several ways and most Canadians are deficient in it; certainly inactive elderly shut-ins like Anne almost always are.
4. I ordered a powerfully anabolic bone drug called *teriparatide* (it acts a bit like a bodybuilder's steroids but for the bone, not the muscle) for her to take afterwards too.

At the first post-op visit at three weeks, it all looked great and Anne was very happy. Her pain drug dose was already lower than it had been in years. I measured the X-rays, and sure enough, I had realigned her by 30 degrees. But she was still 20 degrees off from the 10 degrees' malalignment that's the upper limit of normal, and so risks remained high.

At her second post-op visit at two months, she still felt great but had crumbled her T10 despite my screw fixation there, and that bone had tilted forward by about 10 degrees. How? Sure enough, despite everything she had been through and despite all my preaching and nagging and begging and explaining how delicate her situation was, she admitted to bending forward to pick stuff up. Even with the brace on, that was enough to overload her osteoporotic spine and fracture again. You can only do so much to protect people from themselves.

I was not happy. I didn't yell, but I gave her one hell of a lecture.

At four months and six months, the new fracture had healed and she came out of the brace. Some gentle rehab exercises started.

At a year she was happy. Still deformed by 30 degrees in her low back and another 10 at T10, still having backache and some muscle spasm and taking some drugs, but much better than she had been in years and happy. No walker, no cane! We parted company.

SPINE CRIMES

The error in surgical spine care is almost always to do too little once we make the decision to operate. Here one might ask why I didn't realign and fuse her L3/L4 at the very first surgery, but at that point it would have been hard to justify a bigger, riskier and more expensive operation when we know how good the results of discectomy for sciatica are. I had thought about it, and we had talked about it, but if something had gone wrong with more surgery at that point, I'd have been unable to defend it.

But that second discectomy, done with a full laminectomy, was biomechanically a very high-risk thing to do. Unfortunately, the surgical literature doesn't focus on nuances of technique much and says only that a simple discectomy (regardless of technique, that is with or without laminectomy) for repeat hernia is as good in relieving sciatica as adding a fusion, so my colleague could defend himself in court if it ever came to that. Sadly, that literature doesn't look at all the other issues around recurrent disc hernia like spine alignment, balance and stability that can present in patients with advanced degenerative disc disease, like Anne. So the elementary surgeon thinks he's doing the right thing in a complex case. That's a spine crime.

As for the dynamic duo who did the malaligned multilevel fusion, in my ideal world, surgeons who are not dedicated solely to spine care and surgery would be limited to doing only what the board certification exams in orthopedics and neurosurgery expect them to be able to do — take out a first-time disc hernia, do a laminectomy or a simple one-level fusion. Sadly, they aren't.

Chapter 13
Melinda the Active Retiree

Whose spine infection was cured but not early enough to prevent her disability.

Melinda was a fine community-minded woman in her late 60s when I met her, retired and keeping busy as a volunteer, driving people to medical appointments when they needed help with transportation. Nice lady.

Her low back pain came on out of the blue a year before we met, just a backache that started one midday as she sat waiting for a client in her car. It was on and off for a few days and then suddenly it was on all the time, and it built intensity rapidly. Within a month she wasn't working and was barely able to move around the house.

She'd gone to her family doctor about it several times. The GP asked about sciatic symptoms and whether her bowels and bladder were working normally (they were), examined her briefly and told her that acute backache was common and almost always got better within a few weeks.

What's *acute?* we (and Melinda) might ask. Literally the word means *something that just happened right now or very recently.* In backache, most literature calls anything symptomatic for less than six weeks *acute;* longer than that and it's *chronic.*

I think six weeks is way too short a time to get excited about. A badly sprained ankle might easily hurt you for that long. We shouldn't be jumping to operate in spine care unless the pain is very severe or escalating or unorthodox in its presentation, putting up what we call red flags. At six weeks the patient should only be trying meds and seeing physios and chiros and very likely getting better.

But Melinda's back pain kept getting worse. She often felt warm and sweaty with it but never had a fever. Growing doses of pain meds didn't help. When she reached the point where she was having trouble getting out of bed, her family took her to the local ER where the experience mirrored a family doctor visit.

At a second ER visit the doctor helpfully suggested they buy a plastic bedpan from the pharmacy so she didn't have to get up to the bathroom. The third-visit ER guy finally took an X-ray that didn't show much, and then after two days lying on a stretcher in the ER, Melinda got an MRI scan that showed a discitis infection in her L5/S1 disc space.

THE DIAGNOSIS

Spinal infections can be horrible things. In the global lexicon of medical diagnoses these are so rare that many doctors will never see a case. Even in dedicated spine care hospitals they were uncommon until about a decade ago, when for some unclear reason the frequency of this plague skyrocketed around the world. It used to be that we'd see a case every other month or so at my hospital, but today we might have two or three cases on the ward at the same time.

There are three basic types of spine infection. First, going from front to back through your spine, a disc space infection, *discitis*, is likely one of the most painful things a person can suffer. The patient with untreated raging acute discitis is literally afraid to even move in bed. These patients hold their whole body rigidly as they try to minimize disc pressure and control their pain. Sometimes pus can rupture out of the disc space into the neurological canals behind it to cause paralysis, into the chest causing pneumonia, into the abdomen damaging muscles and causing abdominal infection or even into the bloodstream causing septicemia, commonly called blood poisoning. That can lead to shock, organ failure, delirium and even death.

Second, in the "middle" of your spine, infection of the neurological canals, or *spinal epidural abscess* (SEA), also causes exquisite pain and can progress to paralysis.

Third, infections of the bony posterior facet joints — *facet pyarthrosis* — are another potential source of intense pain. They can erode the bones to destabilize the whole structure of the spine and cause crippling deformity, spread into the back muscles to destroy them or rupture into the neurological elements causing paralysis.

These rare infections can happen to anybody but there seem to be two major high-risk groups. One is active IV drug users (IVDUs). Dirty needles can transmit bacteria into the bloodstream easily, and those bacteria commonly anchor in the spine. This is what programs that dispense clean needles to drug users are all about preventing, among other things. The second risk group is less accepted and more loosely defined, but certainly what I see in practice suggests that the patient with a degenerated spine and multiple common illnesses, like diabetes and high blood pressure and heart disease, is at accelerated risk. We almost never see an otherwise healthy-looking spine in a healthy person present with an infection.

These infections are never small things. The disc is the single biggest structure in our body that has no artery supplying blood to it, so antibiotics don't get to it well and treatment with high-dose IV antibiotics has to be continued for months. Ditto with infections in bone. These patients will commonly have a special long-term IV (a PICC) inserted after surgery that stays in after they go home from hospital and home care nurses come in daily for months to administer the antibiotics — that's pricey! Some cases may have to stay in hospital for their own safety, clogging up beds for months.

Most spine infections can be treated successfully with drugs when we catch them early. Even a disc completely dissolved away by infection often calcifies and fuses to recreate a stable anatomy of the spine. These patients do fine, much like most people after a surgical disc fusion that might be done for a number of indications.

But too often these infections are neglected. Frequently, and even despite extreme pain or neurological symptoms, these infections don't cause a high fever or sweatiness and doctors who are unfamiliar with the problem don't recognize it. Infection can slowly dissolve away the structure of your spine to cause a painful instability or compress the neurological bits enough to cause paralysis. That's when spine surgeons like me might have to go to work. We can restore the structure and commonly relieve the pain, but if you're paralyzed, you're usually going to stay that way. There's no cure for that degree of neurological damage.

THE "SUCCESSFUL" TREATMENT

When the radiologist interpreting the MRI diagnosed Melinda's infection, the ER consulted Medicine to get the patient admitted. Medicine consulted the infectious disease (ID) service for advice on best antibiotics, and so on, in a chain of care. All of these people depend on the radiologist to report the scan properly. Many don't actually look at the scan because they don't have to in order to do their work.

In this case that challenged system initially worked well. ID advised that three months' treatment with a specific IV antibiotic would do the job. There's a neat, low-tech and very inexpensive way to assess whether the antibiotics are working early on, using a blood test called the *C-reactive protein (CRP) level.* The CRP is a very nonspecific indicator of inflammatory activity in the patient's system. Just about any illness or injury will kick it up, but with healing it drops rapidly, responding sometimes within hours. Melinda's CRP dropped steadily for several days; correspondingly her pain decreased a lot and after a week or so when she was mobile enough, home she went with her PICC.

Home care nurses came in several times a day to administer those antibiotics, daily for the usual three months. The CRP dropped steadily and was settled at normal levels by just six weeks.

At three months, both an MRI scan and the CRP confirmed the infection had been defeated, so the PICC was removed and the patient was discharged from care.

AFTERMATH

There was only one teensy weensy little problem. Melinda was still hurting at this point. Nobody had asked about her pain; that's not part of the treatment algorithm for infections, is it?

Melinda hurt *a lot*. Whenever she moved. In fact she had hobbled into her follow-up appointment at the ID clinic with a walker and had needed a wheelchair for the long trek from the parking lot into the building. The ID doctor noticed, and she reassured Melinda that her pain could be expected to settle quickly now that the infection was cured. She was in bad shape because she had been so ill for so long — "Try some physio!"

Try some physio? Just getting on and off the toilet was still torture. She felt a deep grinding shear in her back whenever she changed position from sitting to standing or even lying down. She didn't expect physio would be very realistic but she did sign up. Her son helped her hobble in and out of the local clinic a half dozen times where she'd lie on a stretcher while a muscle stimulator machine was applied to her legs. Didn't do much.

After a month of this she gave up and called the infectious disease doctor's clinic only to be told that her case was closed and she should see her family doctor.

The family doctor, knowing the infection had been cleared, prescribed some pain meds. Again nothing worked, even narcotics.

After three months of all that Melinda was wheelchair-bound and completely dependent on her son who had taken a leave of absence from work to look after her. She convinced her family doctor to order a new MRI.

The scan report said there was no infection. At the office visit where her GP presented that good news, his patient broke down and cried in despair — if she was so healthy, why was she in such pain, why couldn't she stand or move or walk? The family doctor asked if she would consider referral to spine care and potential surgery, and she agreed.

At the spine clinic Melinda couldn't be examined properly because she couldn't stand up. Any attempt to move her on the stretcher caused a shriek of pain. The nurse clinician seeing her was able to gently reach around under her and find that she wasn't actually very tender to gentle manual pressure applied to her back, despite her back muscles being in rigid spasm. He was able to determine that there was no paralysis and her leg muscles were in fact quite strong despite everything she'd been through. He read the report of the scan confirming the infection had been cured and presented the case to the clinic's surgeon as nonoperative. The surgeon agreed; with no neurological deficit and no neurological compression or infection in the scan, there was nothing to be done here. He suggested referral to the chronic pain clinic for pain-relieving injections.

Back at the family doctor's office, Melinda was in tears again. The family doctor called me to ask if I'd provide a second opinion, and I was able to see her in my clinic a week later.

The scan didn't show any evidence of infection. But neither did it show any evidence that the infected disc space had calcified. There was no fusion. What it did show to the educated eye was evidence of terrible instability. The lower half or so of her L5 vertebra had been ground away and rounded off to match the top of her sacrum, the bone of the pelvis immediately below it. There was a big sterile fluid gap where the lower half of the L5 vertebra should be. The posterior facet joints correspondingly were fractured and eroded away at that level.

In X-rays and an MRI taken with her lying down flat on her back, things looked very much like they did in the scan, no great surprise there. Standing X-rays can be helpful in a complex spine case, but we couldn't do that here because Melinda just hurt too much. The best I could do towards getting her erect was to ask her to pant with the pain while they elevated the head of the stretcher into a seated position where an X-ray showed the L5/S1 disc space collapsed completely and the L5 vertebra slid forward on the sacrum by about a half inch. This spine was completely unstable!

How do we define spinal stability? Good question. Most mechanical systems — and your spine is a mechanical support structure after all — are not completely rigid but designed to be a bit wobbly, they have some "give" under stress. A flagpole waves back and forth in a stiff wind, even skyscrapers warp back and forth a bit, but they're stable to such stress and within the confines of a limited amount of "give" or wobble. A hurricane might overwhelm the flagpole, but thankfully skyscrapers are designed to be stronger.

Surgeons are fundamentally simple people. We like black-and-white definitions of what wiggle or malalignment would be acceptable in a spine, or not. There's a big volume of biomechanical research on this point. Classically we talk about so many millimeters of slide or degrees of angulation, but what's in the lab doesn't always translate very well to the clinic. The best definition of spinal instability comes from the bible of biomechanics, White and Panjabi's book, *Clinical Biomechanics of the Spine*, and it's a holistic one: " . . . the inability of the spine to support physiological loads without progressive deformity, neurological compression or unrelenting pain." Too many spine surgeons are not familiar with this book, and the field of biomechanics generally.

Melinda fit this classic definition. So what to do? We wouldn't be treating infection here; we'd be treating *instability*. In spine care, we do that with a fusion operation. Immediately many physicians panic with conflict at the concept here, fearing that our cure would only be making the original problem worse by potentially introducing a new implant-related infection. Fusions generally require screws and whatnot to be implanted into the spine. Bacteria like to stick to the surface of metal implants and antibiotics can't get to them well there, so implant-related infections can be very difficult, sometimes impossible, to cure. In hip and knee replacement surgery done with massive stainless-steel implants in leg bones known to have poor blood flow, they can even lead to amputations!

Spines are a little different. In the majority the infected spine is a high-blood-flow and high-oxygen-tension environment, and our implants are not made of stainless steel (like joint replacements) but titanium alloy. Bacteria don't stick to titanium very well. So we should be able to treat spine infections surgically. And we can. We proved that with good-quality research in the early history of implant spine surgery. But very few physicians know it, even many "trained" spine surgeons and certainly (at least, in my experience) most infectious disease people.

Back to Melinda. Her spine was unstable because that lower disc had dissolved away and not been fused. She needed the collapsed disc realigned and stabilizing implants and fusion bone grafts inserted there with screw fixation to secure things temporarily while the bone healed, a process that commonly takes at least three to four months. There's a long list of technical options as to how we can accomplish that, but that's the essence of it.

It's not rocket science. The afternoon after her surgery, when as her surgeon I made ward rounds, I found her standing at the bedside talking to a friend and asking to go home. I kept her in hospital for two days of routine post-op antibiotics and to be sure that culture swabs we had harvested during surgery were as sterile as they had looked to be, and they were. At six weeks she was doing fine and off narcotics for the first time in a year. She didn't show for her next appointment so I called her, only to learn she was just too busy with her life and the work of driving cancer patients to and from the hospital to come to the clinic — and that was fine.

SPINE CRIMES

A serious spine crime was narrowly averted here. If Melinda's family doctor hadn't been caring enough to get his patient a second opinion, she'd still be in pain and largely wheelchair-bound. Not because she'd been treated by bad doctors, but simply because most doctors today don't get enough spine care education.

Spine problems can be obvious, but sometimes they're not. And, as we'll see in the next chapter, sometimes symptoms are attributed to the *obvious* problem when it isn't the *important* problem.

Chapter 14
Max the Mechanic

When backache isn't just backache.

I n my experience, heavy equipment mechanics are almost always the nicest people. Realistically, their work is more life-and-death than mine on a daily basis. Trucks run off the road, cranes topple, loads shift dangerously. These guys have to be calm, cool and thorough. And lucky.

Max at age 60 was a lucky guy. That's when he met his surgeon, after a load shifted on one of his job sites and a crate fell to the ground, striking a glancing blow to Max's head and shoulder before driving six inches into the ground. He regained consciousness in the ER wearing a neck brace, with eight stitches in his shoulder. A surgeon was standing at a computer terminal next to him describing to his students what turned out to be two different broken bones in the neck. Max's neck. As Max realized what was going on, his blood pressure shot up, but as he heard the surgeon say the golden words " . . . should do fine in a collar . . ." he calmed quickly.

Your head weighs as much as a bowling ball, and on average, it takes a minimum of about three months for weight-bearing fractures to stably heal. Max wore that collar like it was his religion for that long, 24/7/365. Missing work, he swallowed his pride and collected workers' compensation benefits to pay the bills. His neck was stiff when the collar came off but it didn't hurt much, and his surgeon taught him some simple stretches. Within a month he was back on the job as good as ever.

The only thing that bothered him was that he had to get up once or twice during the night to pee, but Max had had that issue for some years before his accident. Sixty-year-old men commonly develop a benign overgrowth of the prostate gland called *BPH*, or benign prostatic hyperplasia, which sees us running to the bathroom to pee every few hours. Max had discussed it with his doctor who, after examining him, screened him for prostate cancer with a PSA blood test and checked his kidney function the same way. Everything was fine; he just had to live with it.

But about a year after the accident his bladder started to act up; not once or twice but three or four times a night he was up. Blood tests again, all OK. Six months later it was a bigger problem; he was dribbling a lot and really running to the bathroom, as well as feeling numb down there. He wasn't getting the erections he'd like either. So he was sent to a urologist and the bloodwork came out OK again. The urologist prescribed a drug to shrink the prostate and some Viagra.

He liked the Viagra and it worked well, but that other drug didn't. He got more and more numb and the numbness started to spread down his legs into his feet and up towards his waistline, and his legs started to feel rubbery. His backache got worse and he found himself stooping a lot because he was more comfortable that way. He spoke to his family doctor about it and was sent to see a physiatrist.

After examining Max, the specialist didn't find much except numbness. His leg muscles were strong and his reflexes were normal. Diabetes can cause neuropathy — nerve damage that numbs the legs — so he was sent for a nerve test. The physiatrist was aware that spinal cord compressions can do the same thing so he was also sent for MRI scans of his entire spine. The nerve test was fine, but the MRIs showed disturbingly advanced degeneration throughout his spine.

Disc degeneration is a very common thing. If we take people who have never had backache a day in their lives in off the road and scan them, the odds are roughly the patient's age in years that the scan will show worn discs, even to the point of some spinal stenosis or malalignment. If they're asymptomatic, nobody should care!

There are only five well-defined risk factors that accelerate anatomic disc degeneration; these don't necessarily impact pain or the chance of disability but the anatomic degeneration itself. They are: 1) being super overweight; 2) doing physical work with a lot of bending and lifting; 3) frequent exposure to heavy motor vibrations like driving a large truck with a diesel engine; 4) smoking; and 5) high levels of personal stress. Max had all five. So there was no surprise in these scans.

When the physiatrist saw that the nerve test showed no degeneration of the sensory nerves, he knew that pretty much settled that question, but he also knew that the EMG that tests motor nerve function was very insensitive. Numbness from the waist down is a classical clinical complaint with spinal cord compression. He himself didn't feel qualified to read the scan directly, so after suggesting that Max use a cane because he was so unsteady on his feet, he referred him to the surgeon at the local workers' compensation spine clinic.

Workplace injuries have unique implications to wage earners and the families they support, so most countries have some sort of workers' compensation system that not only provides support to injured workers but can accelerate their diagnosis and care. It's a "second tier" of health care that's accepted even in Canada. Back injuries are just about the most common industrial injuries and so the back clinic is an obvious component of this system.

At the back clinic, Max was scheduled to see a surgeon who could offer surgery if need be. These surgeons are trained to evaluate disability in a narrowly defined legal way and so they spend a lot of time doing detailed reports and paperwork. They can operate too but most don't. (If they were great operators, they wouldn't be working in clinics pushing paperwork all day, would they?) In many of these facilities, they are so busy they are assisted by physician amplifiers who have some of the same training in disability evaluation (in the States a physician's assistant, or in Canada perhaps a nurse practitioner). None of these people get the deep clinical experience that comes from looking after people over time as one might in an office-based surgical practice.

Max's experience at the clinic wasn't great. After a long walk from the parking lot and hobbling into the place with his cane, Max was given a number of forms to fill out and spent a half hour in the busy waiting room ticking boxes on those forms, answering questions about his injury and symptoms and what he could or couldn't do physically since. Then he was introduced to a woman who identified herself as a nurse practitioner and examined him for about 10 minutes. Then the doctor arrived, said hello without identifying himself and spoke to the nurse practitioner about the case for a minute. He eyeballed Max's MRI for all of about 10 seconds and told him that there was nothing more to be done and that he should be happy with the 20 percent disability pension income the compensation board would be awarding him. Obviously he could never work again — how does a mechanic work with a cane?

Max asked a few questions. He'd been hurt; couldn't he be fixed? The doctor said no, we can't fix a back where every single disc is badly worn out. Max said his family doctor and the physiatrist had told him that he'd likely had disc degeneration for years, maybe decades. So why did he suddenly have such pronounced symptoms? Could that much more disc degeneration have happened in one short year since the accident? The doctor had no answer for that.

A month later when the compensation board report came through, Max's family doctor couldn't believe it. By this point Max needed a walker to hold himself up — how could there be nothing to cause this sudden neurological deficit? He was able to get his patient a second opinion from an independent surgeon.

That was a different experience. After a solid 10 minutes of answering this doctor's questions about what he could and couldn't do because of his pain, the guy asked Max to take a finger and point to where it hurt. Up to this point nobody had ever asked him to do that. Max touched the *top* of his low back, not the bottom where much generalized back pain occurs. This doctor asked him to get up and walk around, poked his back a bit, had him bend and twist in six different directions and even touch his toes. *What is this, gymnastics class?* Then the doctor had him climb onto the exam room stretcher to examine him neurologically — he could barely do it. The surgeon tried to explain that all the gymnastics were part of a properly thorough spine exam. *Suuure. Nobody else made me do all that; hope you're getting your jollies.*

Then this surgeon put Max's MRI scan up on a computer monitor and showed him not only how each and every disc was quite worn across the length of his low back, but also the one single place where his spinal cord was actually squished by a combination of disc bulge and spinal stenosis, at the T10/T11 level. That's just above the top of your low back, right where Max had pointed. Duh. Surgery could help that. But . . .

The doctor wasn't happy and explained that because Max had by this point been symptomatic for many months, he almost certainly would never fully recover. Most people know that spinal cords are delicate and that *full* paralysis is permanent. However, Max learned that neurological tissue can tolerate being pinched or compressed a great deal as spurs might slowly grow over months and years. Eventually though, compression reaches a point where squished nerve cells are dying off in a big way and symptoms start. Generally speaking, those nerve cells keep dying off unless they're decompressed. How well the patient might recover after surgery depends a great deal on how long they have been symptomatic and how badly off they are to start with. Bladder function loss was the worst sign of how advanced his condition was.

Nonetheless the surgeon suggested something should be done to at least stop things from getting worse — but there were risks. The surgery could even cause paralysis! The decompression operation would weaken the structure of his spine, and because Max was such a big guy and did such heavy work, the surgeon wanted to put some strengthening screws in and do a fusion at the same time. *Sheesh, that's gonna hurt!*

Max wasn't ready to decide so he didn't at first but made another appointment with the surgeon for the next week. He went home and spoke with his wife. They wrote down a lot of questions, including if this was a surgical case, why had the radiologist and the compensation doctor insisted it wasn't? A week later the surgeon answered all their questions and Max agreed to surgery.

Surgery was scheduled quickly and it worked well. Max woke up sore from the cut but relatively pain free, with most of the numbness gone and his legs feeling stronger. He'd had a bladder catheter inserted, which the doctor explained was routine for the surgery and the nurses removed it the next morning. He felt the need to go to the bathroom and had a nice big pee around two o'clock and was fine after that.

Max went home from the hospital the second day after surgery and was sore enough from the incision to need some mild narcotics a few times a day for a month. By the time that "pain of the cut" was past, he felt pretty good on his feet so he went to see his boss and asked if his old job was still open. His boss just about kissed him.

Max handled his old job easily. Stiff and sore after work, sure, but he was a 60-year-old guy and had been stiff and sore after work for a long time. Legally, he couldn't be rehired full-time until the comp claim was closed so back he went to the compensation board clinic. He saw the same doctor he'd seen there before, who didn't seem to remember him at all and buried his nose in the case notes to avoid making eye contact. He couldn't explain why he'd been willing to leave Max half paralyzed and seemed reluctant to close the claim file, but when Max explained what had happened, he did.

Max wasn't happy. He'd been really lucky that his family doctor sent him for a second opinion — but what if he hadn't? After some time, he realized that the fool of a compensation board doctor might do the same thing to the next guy, so he wrote a letter about it to the compensation board office and told them they should fire the guy. He doesn't know what came of it.

SPINE CRIMES

Inadequate initial assessment of this case led to missed diagnosis, unnecessary disability and suffering and could even have resulted in paralysis if Max's GP had not been alert enough to solicit a second opinion. Sadly, too many people like Max fall through the cracks in the system not because doctors are uncaring but mostly because they're not well trained in spine care. Which leads to common spine crimes:

1. **Inadequate medical history:** Asking patients to check boxes on a long form and to answer a few cursory questions is simply not enough. If the patient is in pain, it's critical to ask pointed, probing questions about what they can or can't do because of it, where it is in the body (ask them to point to it with a finger!) and what happens with activity — is it better or worse?

2. **Inadequate physical exam:** If the patient says they can't stand and walk, have them try to stand and walk! You need to see what's going on mechanically, what causes them pain, what they can and can't do.

3. **Tunnel vision:** Assuming the work injury is just a work injury. If a patient is in pain, particularly with sudden onset, you need to dig deeper.

Happens all the time. Too many never get that correct second opinion.

Chapter 15
Noronha the Nurse

> *A narrow escape from a crooked artery
> in the neck.*

N oronha was a very successful career nurse who had worked her
way up through the ranks, starting as a scared kid in her 20s and
retiring from her last roles as a senior nurse manager and educator
when she qualified for her maximum pension in her mid-50s. But she
never wanted to leave her work totally behind her. She really loved
teaching and so she contracted out to a firm that managed hospitals
and in her second career was regularly being sent around the world to
share her skills. She missed the grandkids but otherwise it was a ball!

Approaching 60, she'd been lucky. Many if not most people
have plenty of aches and pains at that point in life (like I do!) but
mostly she didn't. So it was unusual for the odd little kink she'd
noticed in her neck during a return flight home from overseas to
last through to deplaning. And the next day, and the day after that.
And the next, and the week after that. Her neck was a bit stiff,
and after a while, pain spread down to the top of her left shoulder
too. She tried hot showers, Tylenol and Advil, and nothing made
a difference. The constant nagging ache bugged her so she saw her
family doctor who said she'd not found much on examination, then
sent her to physio and ordered some X-rays.

Two days later the doctor's office called and asked her to come back in. The GP wore a worried expression, told her there was a lot of advanced arthritis and a partial dislocation or subluxation in her neck, and gave her a copy of the two-page radiology report. Noronha didn't want to believe it. How could it be so bad? She'd never been sore a day in her life before this. She needed convincing and asked to see the actual X-rays, but the doctor's office wasn't equipped to do that for her. Her doctor was concerned and said she needed an MRI and should see a surgeon; that subluxation meant her spinal cord might be at risk. She also wanted her to start wearing a rigid neck support collar 24/7/365.

Yeah right, you try wearing a hard neck support collar all day, all night. First up, Noronha, who was extremely familiar with the potential for health care screwups, wanted her X-rays repeated. Maybe the films reported here weren't actually hers and she'd been mixed up with somebody else. Doc hadn't thought of that. Good idea, off to X-ray again.

Same report. This time Noronha asked for a digital copy of her images on a disc and tossed it into her computer at home. *Holy crap!* She immediately put the collar on. Her whole neck was collapsing forward. It looked like her chin was heading for her breastbone.

Her MRI followed a short while later, by which time the pain went to both shoulders and extended down to her right elbow. Her shoulders felt heavy, and she was having trouble lifting her arms enough to do her hair. Her right hand felt a bit odd too, somewhat numb and her fingers were stiff and awkward. She was having trouble putting in her earrings and texting. The report said, "High-grade spinal cord compression with myelomalacia at C4/C5. Surgical consult recommended."

Oh shit. Noronha thought she remembered that myelomalacia meant scarring in the spinal cord and that was a bad thing. Dr. Google confirmed it and she started calling that surgeon's office every day, pushing for an earlier appointment than the one she'd been given.

The office appointment with the surgeon wasn't a good time. The secretary snarled at her, *Oh it's you!* Apparently calling the busy important doctor's office before your appointment wasn't appreciated. The waiting room was jammed. An hour and a quarter after her appointment time, the surgeon saw her and spent all of five minutes getting her story and glancing at the scan on-screen. He told her she needed an operation at C4/C5 to correct the subluxation, decompress her spinal cord and stabilize her neck with screws and a bone graft fusion. This could be done with surgery on the front of the neck or from the back. He said the posterior approach was best; the operation would be a laminectomy on C4 and screw fixation across C4/C5. It was so complicated he couldn't do it alone; he'd need assistance from a second surgeon. He could book it in a few weeks. She'd need to stay in her collar for a few months after surgery, until the bone knit. Noronha felt dizzy with the stress, and terrified, but agreed to book it.

Surgery was hell. The anesthetist said she couldn't insert the breathing tube normally because Noronha's neck was so bent out of shape, so she had to do an awake intubation. Noronha swizzled an anesthetic mouthwash until she couldn't feel her tongue and was given some light sedative drugs, but she was fully awake and aware as the anesthetist snaked a two-foot-long fibreoptic endoscope down her throat before sliding the big breathing tube in over it. Only then was she knocked out. Noronha had been told that she wouldn't remember the intubation afterwards, but when she woke she did, and her throat was so sore she could barely speak or swallow. For a day she was drooling because she couldn't even swallow her spit.

The big cut on the back of her neck was killing her. She was sore as hell just above her ears and across the top of her skull, where, she later learned, her head had been bolted into a special metal clamp that held it rigidly in place during the delicate spine operation.

But the kink in her neck was gone, ditto the pain in her shoulder. Her right hand was working normally again, and so she put up with these post-op symptoms and thanked the surgeon for helping her when he discharged her a few days later.

Two months in the collar was OK, but her neck was stiff as a board, so the surgeon sent her to physio. She was a bit sore after physio, but she learned that this was expected at first and she should "work through the pain." It would settle in a month or two. She tried. It didn't settle. After a few months the after-physio soreness was just as severe and just as constant as the original kink in her neck had been; in fact, it felt just about the same. So she called the surgeon's office for an appointment.

And didn't get one. She was told that because she had already had her "successful" surgery, there was nothing more the surgeon could do for her; if she still had pain, she should ask the family doctor to send her to the pain clinic. Noronha wasn't impressed with the level of professionalism here, but what could she do?

The pain clinic was very accommodating. They saw her within a week and she learned that she would need regular bimonthly nerve block injections for the rest of her life to "manage" her chronic pain. Insurance would pay for it and there was no co-pay, isn't that nice? *Shit. OK, let's go.*

Fifteen injections later she was no better. Her hand was all wonky again, and now her leg too. Again the surgeon's office refused a second re-referral from her family doctor, so she asked to be sent to another surgeon for a second opinion. That surgeon wanted a CT scan and another MRI before he'd see her. *Arrogant bastard, WTF?* When the new scans had been done, in she went.

SECOND OPINION

The second surgeon's office was different. There was a clean, modern, quiet waiting room with not a lot of patients. *Who is this guy? How good can he be if nobody's coming to see him?* Still she waited almost an hour after her appointment time to be seen. During the wait, she was sent for some weird X-rays of her neck. She was sitting up rather than lying down with the collar off, and they even had her flex and extend her neck as much as she could. Back in the waiting room she could see the second surgeon peering at his computer screen, looking at scans and reports. She started to have doubts. *Why should it take so long to figure out her scans? Was this guy even smart enough to give her an opinion?*

At the interview, he grilled her for a good 15 minutes about her symptom history and her operation. Asked for a lot of details about her symptoms going away after surgery, and how they came back. Were they the same or different? Then he did an odd thing: asked her to stand up and walk a bit. Again, *WTF, the first guy never did that.* He spent another 15 minutes examining her neck, shoulders, arms, hands, legs, feet, you name it. He asked her why she had screws just in one side of her neck and not both — she didn't know that, had no idea.

The second surgeon showed her the X-rays and scans. He explained that her spine had continued to collapse dramatically since the first surgery. It was so bent now you could see in the MRI scan how the spinal cord was pulled forward against the bones of her neck. She needed much more done to get her better aligned and stable. The first surgery had addressed only the C4/C5 level and there was a lot more going bad everywhere here.

OK. So, why? Had the first surgery destabilized something?

Yes. A little. But likely as not, it had also been caused by the cumulative damage to her spinal cord from the advanced arthritis.

The second surgeon explained that the bowling ball mass of the head is not balanced squarely atop the neck that supports it but is offset forward a bit — that's why if we relax our neck muscles the head falls forward. Noronha's arthritis was everywhere; not only had every single one of the six discs that support the head in the front of the neck completely collapsed to the point where bone was rubbing on bone, but the bony facet joints in the back of the neck that create stability were eroded too. That's why she had slipped out of joint at C4/C5. Now she was slipping out of joint at C5/C6, just below the old surgery, too. Fortunately her spinal cord was not pinched there this time, but it was being pulled forward and stretched so much that her neurological symptoms had returned from just that.

He said the Gore angle in her neck was 30 degrees, which was bad, and the arthritis in her neck had deformed her so much that her head was about two inches anterior to (in front of) where God had designed it to be. Getting her straight would best be done with an operation on the front of her neck. *All* those worn discs and bone spurs would have to be removed and the collapsed disc spaces elevated, bone grafts inserted to support them, and a great big metal plate screwed down over it all to hold it for the months it takes to heal. This would be a major operation that might take all day, and she'd likely have to go into ICU for a while afterwards.

How can my neck be so arthritic and worn out? A year ago I was traveling and teaching and doing just fine!

The second surgeon told her that wear-and-tear arthritis in the neck is very common, so much so that some research studies show roughly half of all 50-year-olds are so arthritic they have some spinal cord compression — without symptoms! Careful physical examination of those asymptomatic people finds that about 10 percent in fact have some abnormal neurological findings that they haven't noticed.

That's a challenge for spine surgeons: should surgery be done to prevent things going bad in the future? The verdict is no. Similar population research studies followed these people forward in time for a decade and found that only 20 percent would develop important neurological deficits in that decade. So current best practice is to explain the situation clearly and teach the patient what the early symptoms of trouble are, so that if things do go bad, they can zoom off to their doctor and have it dealt with right away.

The most common early symptom of a spinal cord compression is numbness throughout the fingers and hands that's constant and doesn't change with positioning of the wrist. Some people will have troubles with fine motor control, a change in handwriting or trouble texting or doing up their buttons for a short while even before that. (Recall that Noronha's hands had been numb and awkward for a year before this all happened. Her doctor had told her she had arthritis and suggested some Advil that hadn't helped.)

Why did you ask me about the screws? Is putting them on only one side unusual? Would more screws have made things stronger and prevented this?

The second surgeon hesitated again. He said yes, one side is unusual. He said the first surgeon's OR report described a failed attempt to put screws on both sides. On one side, they would not hold tight in the bone (no explanation why) so he'd removed them before they could come loose. Then the second surgeon showed Noronha her pre-op scans, which revealed an abnormal artery in her neck.

Two of the four blood vessels that bring blood to the brain actually run *inside* the vertebral bones; the vertebral arteries are within millimeters of where the screws go, so damage there is always a risk. (*He never told me that . . .*) Rarely these arteries can be abnormally kinked or swollen. That creates a larger hole in the bone where they are situated, and screws don't hold very well when they are drilled into a hole. The second surgeon explained that Noronha was very lucky the artery hadn't been damaged by the attempted screw fixation there. If it had, she might have suffered a major stroke or even bled out.

He said yes, more screws might have been better. Her operation had involved laminectomies at two of the seven bones in the neck, C4 and C5. Her surgeon had set screws there for strengthening but had not connected those screws to the un-operated, stronger spine above and below. In any mechanical system, if we stiffen a joint, mechanical forces are concentrated alongside it. So Noronha's surgery had created a biomechanical "perfect storm" of increased stress at the surgical site and a weakened connection to the normal anatomy above and below it. A more knowledgeable surgeon would have set screws and done fusion including C3 above and C6 below. Noronha had obviously not been treated by knowledgeable surgeons.

Noronha was horrified about the artery.

Why do such a crazy dangerous thing in the first place?

The second surgeon pointed out that the abnormal artery was not reported by the radiologist who read her scans nor commented on by either the surgeon or his buddy. It seemed that everybody had missed it. That's why it's so important that one's surgeon thoroughly review the scans, which takes more than a few seconds to do properly (now Noronha started to apologize for grumping about her wait at the office today . . .).

Could my original surgery have been done from the front and might that have been any better or safer?

The second surgeon paused. Yes, he informed her, it could have been done that way and maybe it should have been, because working from the front brings both the best shot at realigning a collapsed neck and avoids the problem of weakening the structure that comes with a posterior approach.

He described how, because the head is not balanced directly above the neck, surgery to release the spinal cord by removing posterior structure weakens that neck to the point where, historically, about 30 percent of patients having simple laminectomy in the neck would have the whole thing collapse — like she had. So back in the 1990s it became largely standard to do a screws-and-bone-graft fusion to strengthen the neck at the same time as a decompression, to offset that weakening effect.

Why would a surgeon do a more dangerous and less effective operation than the best one for his patient?

The second surgeon hesitated again. Ignorance, he said. The guy likely just didn't know any better. Ditto his sidekick.

So how do I know that YOU know what you're doing?

The second surgeon told her flat out, you don't. Usually nobody tracks what a surgeon does, and how well or how badly it's done. Any board-certified orthopedic surgeon or neurosurgeon is legally qualified to operate on your spine, but without specialty spine training and a rigorous program of lifelong learning, they likely shouldn't be doing it — just as the generally qualified neurosurgeon shouldn't be doing the most complex "skull base" work, or community orthopedists be treating complex pediatric deformities or bone cancers. The second surgeon then started to list off his specialty training, research, publications and spine society memberships and offered that she could talk to other people he had treated for similar problems. Noronha was reassured — a bit.

Why will I need the ICU?

The second surgeon explained that in operating on the front of the neck, the surgeon has to move all the throat, swallowing and airway structures in there off to one side during the surgery. That retraction can cause a hell of a sore throat and the patient should expect some difficulty swallowing for at least a month; many surgeons advise a soft diet for at least that long. It can cause a temporary change of voice from swelling in the flesh of the neck or the stretching of the nerves to the voice box. These are common issues in surgery addressing just one or two disc levels, which is often accomplished as day surgery — but Noronha's operation was going after *all six discs!* The usual incision is horizontal, roughly paralleling a shirt collar, giving access to at most three disc levels. She would need either two or maybe even three standard incisions or a long vertical slash (which some surgeons try to avoid because it often heals with a very ugly scar).

All that incising and retracting could cause a lot of swelling — potentially enough to squeeze her airway closed. Sometimes at the end of the operation, the anesthetist can see that there's so much swelling it would be unsafe to take the breathing tube out, in which case the patient is discharged to the ICU with the tube on board until the swelling resolves and breathing is safe. With operations on more than three disc levels, even when things go well and we are able to safely wake up and extubate the patient, common practice is to manage the patient in ICU overnight just in case more swelling develops. Many surgeons give their patients steroids for a while after surgery to help with the swelling.

The second surgeon also told Noronha she might even need more than one operation. The strongest possible biomechanical fixation we can apply to the spine in the neck comes from a front-and-back operation that involves implant surgery both anterior and posterior — in fact, two operations in one. He said many surgeons might insist on that for a case like hers but, assuming her neck realigned reasonably well, he thought that she might get away with just the one surgery. Still, she'd certainly have to wear her collar religiously for several months afterwards. He would continue to monitor her with regular monthly X-ray checks until the fusion was healed. If things collapsed, she'd need a posterior revision surgery. She could live with that risk, understanding the issue up front.

REOPERATION

Surgery went great. It did take all day but that collapsed alignment corrected acceptably and the bones in Noronha's neck were hard enough that the screws felt rock solid. Anesthesia did put her into ICU, but she was extubated successfully the next morning with a normal voice and was able to swallow. Her legs and arms felt better that next morning — not perfect, but better. A few days later she went home, still griping about how much she hated her collar.

Noronha's fusions knit and her improved alignment was maintained. Her neurological symptoms of numbness and awkwardness slowly improved over the course of that first year to the point where she wasn't really troubled by the minor residuals at all. The second surgeon had her come into the office periodically for that whole first year, then she had some X-rays done at 18 and 24 months and he reviewed them online so she didn't have to travel to the office. Now she's fine.

SPINE CRIMES

Years later, her first surgeons were still out there legally operating on people. In ignorance. Another spine crime.

Chapter 16
Sarah's Story

When a senior isn't just slowing down.

In her late 70s, Sarah was in a good place in her life. She'd retired from a great job as an administrative assistant to a busy executive a decade earlier, with a nice pension from earlier work as a teacher and a topped-up retirement savings account. She and her husband of almost 50 years could afford to travel. The kids had done well, the grandkids were all in or just out of college and launching into solid careers and she already had one adorable great-grandbaby.

She relished her life because a decade earlier she had come close to losing it all. A bad cold back then had left her with a sore chest and when she was rubbing some ointment on it, she'd felt a lump in her breast. The biopsy was positive for cancer. A surgeon offered lumpectomy, but she'd said no, get the whole thing off. When her lymph nodes were pronounced clean, she was told she didn't need chemo or radiation after all, just a daily tamoxifen pill that blocked some hormone receptor thing and discouraged further cancer growth. *Whew!* She and her husband had booked a tropical vacation that very same day.

Pill or no pill, her cancer doctors insisted they see her regularly for monitoring and she had scans done every so often just to be sure. They were all fine.

ONSET

Ten years on, hours of Christmas baking got her a bit stiff and sore in her neck. All the overhead reaching decorating the tree irritated it more, and after the holiday Tylenol and Advil weren't helping. She'd been thinking about asking her family doctor for a physiotherapy referral but couldn't fit an appointment into her busy schedule.

Her annual cancer check was early in the New Year and when the doctors there asked about her health all she could complain about was that nagging sore neck. The oncologist was concerned because cancer can spread into the spine, and neck or back pain is the most common symptom. This was news to Sarah. He suggested a nuclear medicine scan, a sensitive test to check for cancer spreading to bones, and it was scheduled a week later.

She arrived at the clinic early in the day and was given an IV injection of a radiochemical, which would circulate through her body and concentrate anywhere bone was irritated. The nuclear radiologist explained that *any* little bone irritation from age-related arthritis would be detected, but a cancer would "light up like a fire-cracker" and easily guide treatment.

The drug had to circulate in her bloodstream for a few hours before she could be scanned so they let her go home for a while. When she came back all she had to do was lie flat and very still on a stretcher-thing for about 10 minutes while a big metal scanner was suspended just above her. That was scary but she was able to relax right afterwards when the radiologist told her there was nothing there, just a bit of arthritis in her neck as we might expect. *Phew!*

Her oncologist didn't agree. Because she was having pain at the bottom of her neck and none of the other bits of arthritis that had been found were hurting, he smelled a rat and asked her to have a CT scan as well. That report was also negative and then everybody could really relax.

But Sarah still had pain. Physio didn't help; she went for therapy a few times a week for a month and a half, and nothing changed. Her family doctor recommended massage and Tylenol, but they didn't work either. The nagging pain woke her up once or twice a night when she'd roll over. It seemed to kill her appetite, and she lost about five pounds.

By Mother's Day, she was tiring quickly and feeling unsteady on her feet when she was in the kitchen for a long time preparing one of the great family meals she liked to host. The family doctor wasn't happy so she sent Sarah for an X-ray that didn't show much except a bit of degeneration in her spine, and then she ordered an MRI scan too.

DIAGNOSIS

Three days later the GP called Sarah back into the office and spent an unusual amount of time asking about her pain symptoms and examining her neurologically. When she found how weak Sarah's legs were, she looked concerned. The MRI had found cancer in her upper thoracic spine between the shoulder blades. A Great Big Cancer. The report said it was "massive" and growing forward into her chest and pressing against the back of her heart. Three vertebrae had been quite completely replaced by cancer.

The family doctor had never read a report like this and didn't know if anything could be done. Before her appointment with Sarah, she'd called the oncologist to find out. Oncology said radiation might kill the tumor, but because it was reported to be so big Sarah should see a spine surgeon about it.

The GP told Sarah she had already requested a referral and set up an appointment for her the following week. Sarah's immediate reaction was *Surgery? I'm 70! No thanks, let's do that radiation.* She was adamant, so the family doctor had Sarah and the oncologist talk directly. Oncology convinced Sarah to keep the appointment with the surgeon.

The spine surgeon wasn't happy either. He said this tumor was huge, and he showed her the scan that revealed a big lumpy thing where most of her upper spine was supposed to be. Sarah was shocked and full of questions.

Why didn't this show up on the X-ray?

The surgeon explained that X-rays are very insensitive to spine cancer. Roughly half the bone has to be eroded away by cancer before it can be seen on X-rays. Even "old-fashioned" nuclear medicine isn't very sensitive in spine cases. MRI is known from some obscure Canadian research to detect many spine metastatic cases that would otherwise be missed early on, but that information had somehow never seemed to become mainstream medical knowledge. It was published in the spine literature and not the cancer (oncology) literature. Oops. Also, payors like governments and insurance companies would obviously prefer the inexpensive older test over more expensive MRI imaging. A PET scan is known to be the best "cancer finder" there is, but in many Canadian provinces the state pays for that only in very specific situations, and Sarah's didn't qualify.

Why didn't it show up on the CT scan?

Actually it did — but it was a CT scan of the neck, not the thoracic spine below it where the tumor was, and where Sarah's pain had really focused all along! Knowing where to look, the surgeon could identify some very subtle abnormalities that were likely cancerous, just on the lower edge of the CT scan where the neck blends into the T-spine. Radiology had missed it, perhaps understandably. It was literally on the edge of the scan images the surgeon showed to Sarah.

Why wasn't the scan focused on where it hurt?

No good reason other than the oncologist hadn't asked for it. He'd never asked Sarah to simply take a finger and point to the hurt, assuming the "neck" meant the cervical spine. Often pains below the neck at the top of the shoulder blades (that's the upper thoracic spine) are described as neck pains.

Why hasn't my spine collapsed?

Sarah could barely see any bone in her spine at all in the MRI pictures, but the surgeon explained that almost half of the biomechanical strength of the thoracic spine comes from the rib cage and breastbone attached to it — and they were fine.

Can you cut the cancer out, like we did 10 years ago?

No. OK perhaps more accurately, maybe. Removing something like this would require an extraordinary and very massive operation called an *en bloc resection*. It would involve cutting six ribs (three on each side) away from her spine, dissecting deep into the chest to free the tumor from the back of the heart and the adjacent lungs, doing three laminectomies and gently rotating the cancer around her spinal cord and out of the chest.

Six or eight of the intercostal nerves that went from the spinal cord to the ribs would have to be cut to accomplish this. That would leave her rib cage weak and numb, likely painful, and she'd be short of breath. She'd also need a massive reconstruction operation using custom implants to reassemble her spine. An operation like that might easily be fatal. So maybe let's not.

The surgeon said that Sarah should definitely have surgery, just not *that* surgery. Rather than "going for the cure," he suggested something a bit less aggressive, a palliative operation.

Palliative? Like, I'm going to die now?

Not so; the term *palliative* literally means to relieve symptoms or provide support care. Sarah was palliating her pain when she'd take a pain pill. Surgery for spine metastatic cancer is enormously effective in relieving pain and preventing paralysis, even often reversing neurological deficits when they are present. But spine surgery can almost never *cure* cancer, so she'd now be needing radiation and chemo and all that other bad stuff. Spine metastatic cancer patients generally survive about two years after the diagnosis, though many (especially breast cancer cases, which are usually quite sensitive to radiation) will live much longer than that.

CARE

Sarah didn't know what to do, but when she thought about her family she knew she wanted to enjoy life with them as long as possible, so she agreed to surgery.

Even the palliative procedure was a huge operation, taking all day. Later her surgeon told her that the cardiac room did two hearts in the same amount of OR time, and an orthopedic surgeon replaced five knees.

The spine surgeon had given her an intravenous blood-thickening drug during surgery to decrease the bleeding, but she still lost enough blood to need several units of transfusion in the OR and a few more over the next few days as she recovered in ICU. He was able to remove the back of the tumor as well as both sides and enough anterior tumor to get all the pressure off her spinal cord, preserving all the nerve roots in the process. Then he'd anchored screws into two intact vertebrae above the site and two below, linking them with metal rods that would support the spine while post-op radiotherapy and chemo would hopefully kill off what was left of the tumor.

OUTCOME

Spine surgery works really well most of the time. We can never guarantee the outcome, but we can often give people pretty accurate odds based on the published literature and we see those results in our patients. Sarah got through the surgery without suffering any of the many complications that can come from big surgery in older people and by about six weeks was past the modest pain of the cut and using less pain medicine than she had been using pre-op.

She'd been transferred from acute care to the oncology rehab unit where physios and occupational therapists helped her regain her strength while she had her radiation and started the chemo. She'd lost almost 10 pounds after the surgery — these are very macro-invasive operations and they stimulate the metabolism greatly. Usually the weight comes back, and eventually hers did.

The following Christmas, Sarah was baking and decorating and hosting again. She went on to celebrate with her family for another several years.

SPINE CRIMES

Insensitive diagnostic testing, used for no better reasons than tradition and economy — to save money! That's a spine crime. As are X-rays and scans focused for convenience and tradition rather than directed to "where it hurts." I treat missed cancer cases that present on a delayed basis like this several times every year, and so do most of my colleagues. Sometimes it goes well nonetheless.

But not always.

Chapter 17
Morris's Low Back Miracle

When minimally invasive surgery goes wrong.

M orris couldn't believe it; he thought he was still under anesthetic or dreaming. He was a little sore, a little barfy, had a throbbing headache ... but that searing burn that had tortured his back, right butt cheek and leg for the past four months was *gone*!

A good lawyer doesn't believe anybody up front. There's always backchecking to be done and so he let himself blissfully drift off again — *Why not, these anesthesia drugs were grrreeeaaatttt* — and when his eyes suddenly popped open again, it was real. That sciatica was gone!

He would kiss that surgeon if he could, but senior members of the business community angling for a spot on the hospital board en route to regional politics can't do that.

Morris had the "privacy suite" in the recovery room, as a VIP he warranted that, and so had a bit of control of his surroundings. The bright overhead light was bugging his eyes so he had it turned off. That and getting his contacts back in eased the headache and his stomach settled with some Gravol. A few senior medics and several members of the board he was already friendly with came by as the fog in his head started to clear and the throb of the cut in his low back eased off. No, he couldn't book any golf dates yet, and Doc had told him not to book any big meetings for at least three weeks to be sure he'd be over the worst of his incisional pain and could concentrate properly. He didn't want to make a million-dollar Percocet mistake.

The nurses got annoying really fast as they asked him what his "pain score" was seemingly every two seconds. Really, compared to pre-op he didn't hurt much at all, and when he said "two," they vanished and an orderly came in to help him get dressed. They wouldn't let him walk out of the place so, embarrassed, he sat in a wheelchair as the orderly pushed him through the hospital and out to the parking ramp, where he helped Morris into the car and scored a $20 tip.

At home there was no pain; literally *all* his terrible disabling sciatica was gone. He was all the more motivated to sit on the board of this hospital. What a great place! The nurse practitioner called the next morning to check on him and he sang her boss's praises after giving his pain score as a zero. Headache was an issue but the Tylenol dealt with it, and he was still a bit nauseated from the anesthetic but had some Gravol at home too. His eyes were bugging him for some reason; he had to keep the house lights dim and he had turned down the brightness on his laptop so he could work. That was it. He felt great.

PRELUDE

Four months earlier Morris had had no care in the world other than the big deal that he and his team were working on. He could already retire with Laura any time but loved the cut and thrust of business so he stayed at it, and the details of a major transaction could keep him and his team going for weeks. He had always liked to bring some documents home to reread in bed after a relaxing detox dinner at home. Those "second looks" had helped him avoid a lot of mistakes through the years. It meant that his hands were often full of paperwork on the way to and from the car. One Friday evening, he dropped the keys as he fumbled for them.

As he bent over to pick them up, he'd felt a little *pop!* in his back. Grabbed the keys. Tried to stand back up — and couldn't. Halfway up, the worst pain he'd ever imagined seared out of his rump and down the back of his right leg. *OMG!* He dropped all the papers and fell over. Curling into a ball, he could control the pain but as soon as he started to straighten out he was tortured. Couldn't even crawl back into the car so he called Laura — on his cellphone from the driveway! She couldn't lift him and called an ambulance that took him to the hospital's ER where the MDs drugged him up enough to straighten him out. An MRI scan confirmed he'd had a great big disc hernia at L4/L5 in his low back.

Morris learned most such cases didn't need any surgery. *Good!* Morris wasn't having any surgery; his dad died in an operating room. *No way.* And surgery: *Jeez, surgery would be painful and take me away from the office. I can't afford that right now, can I?*

So he accepted a prescription for the same narcotics he'd been given in the ER and hobbled into the back seat of the Benz, lying flat out across it as Laura drove him home. The ER doctors told him to take it easy through the weekend and likely he'd be much better by Monday.

He wasn't. Couldn't work even from his laptop at home so he had to drop out of the current negotiations. First time in his life he'd ever done that.

Tuesday morning he called his family doctor who proposed a referral to the new acupuncture clinic. He said it was great, all natural so no drugs, and maybe Morris would be able to work again. *Idiot.* The drugs weren't stopping him from working, but the pain that the drugs weren't touching stopped him from thinking straight enough to order lunch!

After mulling it over for about 30 seconds, Morris decided to pull some strings and called the ER director, a physician he'd met at hospital socials, and asked for some help. Sure enough he knew a guy; the senior neurologist in the hospital was good with this stuff and could see him that afternoon.

The neurologist inquired in detail about his symptoms and tortured him through some physical examination. He was frustrated that Morris couldn't lay down on his back for a proper assessment. The only position Morris could get any relief in at all was lying on his side. The neurologist read him the MRI report describing the disc hernia Morris already knew about, told him all the same stuff the ER guy had said and informed him that therapeutic exercises would ease his pain and help him get through it. The chief of physiatry (rehab medicine) would see him tomorrow morning.

Next morning, after yet another night of interrupted sleep, he was at the physiatrist's office. When he was awake, Morris could lie on his side all day in some comfort, but whenever he'd doze off to sleep he'd toss and turn a bit and *Bam!* He'd hurt himself and wake up every hour or so. He was exhausted from lack of sleep. The physiatrist even commented on it, said he looked gray and bagged. *Guy's a genius!*

This doctor spent more time examining him than anybody had so far and was very concerned with some weakness in Morris's ankle; he called that a *drop foot* and explained it was very serious. It could make him stumble, maybe fall even, and if that was happening, he should wear a custom splint called an *AFO*, or ankle-foot orthosis, on his leg to correct it until the nerve damage had time to heal. He wasn't stumbling and so Morris didn't spend $1,500 on a piece of fancy plastic. Morris could concentrate well enough to learn where the guy's physio clinic was located, and then Laura drove him over there for his first treatment.

Physio hurt. A lot. Bend here, stretch there, no pain no gain! Morris left in more pain than he'd had when he got there and didn't fall asleep until 3:00 a.m. after two gins on top of all the useless pills. Tried again the next morning, same story. The next day Laura refused to take him. She was worried and crying.

So they called the physiatrist who was concerned and said he didn't understand it. His program had been number one in the region for years. But OK, nothing works for everybody, and the next step would be a cortisone injection, maybe a series of them.

Cortisone injection? That's a needle, right? But my back already hurts; you want to stick a great big needle in there and hurt me some more?

The physiatrist explained that cortisone is a very powerful steroid anti-inflammatory drug and that it is the inflammation of a pinched nerve that hurts. This made sense and Morris agreed to it. The physiatrist made some calls, explained just who Morris was, and an appointment miraculously became available two hours later.

The nice older chief of anesthesia at the pain clinic was sympathetic and explained that Morris would need a series of three injections, each a week apart, to do the job. Yes, he could do the first right then and there. Within minutes Morris felt a warm flood of numbing relief flow from his buttock down the leg as his pain eased off. It was much easier to hobble back out to the car than it had been to limp into the clinic.

Morris slept through the night, first time since all this began. And the next night. But not the one after that, and on and on as all his pain returned.

He had the same experience the following week, and the week after that.

Enough was enough.

Isn't there surgery for disc hernias?

Morris knew there was. He'd done some personal injuries work at the start of his legal career and worked a few of these cases both for work benefits and malpractice when things had gone wrong . . . "Whoops, when things had gone wrong?" Morris thought about his dad again, and he wasn't too happy about the surgical appointment that the chairman of the board had arranged for him with the hospital's latest hotshot spine surgical recruit.

Morris met a trim younger fellow in his mid-30s or so, just a bit of gray on his temples. He'd trained at all the Best Med Schools and had done the leading spine fellowship, so he was well qualified. There were certificates all over the office that testified to that. He'd passed his boards the first time out, just like Morris had aced his bar exam way back when, so they bonded over that. He showed Morris the scans, which were horrifying, and explained that surgery was highly effective for sciatic pain. It was not so great for backache and Morris might be left with that but it was great for sciatica. Morris told him the story of his dad's post-op heart attack and the surgeon explained that he could do this procedure without a real cut at all; the minimally invasive surgical technology (MIS) was very safe.

How could he do an operation without an incision? The surgeon explained that with guidance from an X-ray fluoroscope in the OR, he would poke a sharp six-inch sterile metal rod called a *K-wire* through the skin and pass it down through the flesh onto the bones bracketing Morris's disc hernia. Then he'd slide a series of dilators over that rod until he had stretched the flesh out to a diameter of about 40 millimeters, about an inch and a half. That was enough of a working channel for the surgeon to drill through the bone and extract not the entire disc but only the damaged bits that were pressing on Morris's nerve, removing just enough tissue to unpinch it. Very safe. Day surgery.

This sounded great and Morris signed up.

REALITY STRIKES

Morris had a very successful surgical experience. At first.

But the headache "from the anesthetic" was an issue. Slowly, it seemed to get worse every day. Tylenol didn't work well for it but those narcotics he'd been prescribed sure did — at first.

Ditto the lights. Laura complained when he had them all turned off and the curtains drawn so he took to wearing his sunglasses in the house. She thought he was nuts.

He really had zero pain but walking around was a bit odd. The top of his foot felt numb in his shoe and he stumbled a lot through the day. At the office, his colleagues also thought the sunglasses were odd. When Morris read through the contract documents they'd worked out without him, he was impressed. That was another worry: *Maybe these guys really don't need me anymore?*

At his surgeon's office two weeks after surgery, a nurse took the one stitch out and the doctor reassured him about his foot, explaining that because the drop foot was "incomplete" it should resolve with time. Could be weeks, could be months, there's no way to predict it, and yes, there was always a small chance it wouldn't recover. No, there was no big need for physical therapy rehab after surgery like this and neither was there a need for repeat visits. He could just go on with his life. That was another big plus of MIS technology: no expensive aftercare.

Two weeks after that he was getting used to the headache and losing the shades. One morning in the shower he noticed a soft bump under the incision on his back and called the surgeon's office. The nurse practitioner explained that even with MIS technique some swelling was normal. *OK, fine.*

A week later as Morris rolled out of bed one morning, he felt a little tug where the incision was and a warm river of clear fluid poured down his back. Headache skyrocketed so he laid back down. It kept coming.

Laura called the ambulance again. He went to the ER again. He had an MRI again. He met a surgeon again.

The on-call surgeon was an older guy who explained that the new scan showed there was a leak of spinal fluid at the surgical site. This was a common complication of spine surgery, when the soft membrane, the dura, surrounding the brain and nerves and containing the spinal fluid might be torn by an instrument — it's a thing in brain surgery too. If leaking was considerable, eventually the fluid could work its way out as it had in Morris's case.

A return to the operating room to repair the leak was advisable because if fluid could leak out, bacteria could potentially work their way in and that could lead to meningitis and all its complications — like septicemia, paralysis, brain damage and even death. The leaking fluid dropped the fluid pressure surrounding the brain; that's why Morris had been having all his headaches and photophobia, the sensitivity to light.

How could this happen with MIS? The surgeon hesitated. He explained that surgery is surgery, big cut or small, and the risks from what we have to do once we're in there are not much different one way or another. MIS is all the rage across all surgeries, but some older surgeons are hesitant about it in spine surgery because it is terribly important to stay oriented in the operating room, to be 100 percent sure where you are within the anatomy and particularly in the tight confines of the spinal canal. With MIS, the limited field of vision one squints at through a 1.5-inch diameter tube that's 6 inches long might detract from that. Most younger surgeons are very enthusiastic about it because in the absence of experience with more classical techniques, they were never taught otherwise. Also it "sells" so well — no patient ever looks forward to having back surgery but most people are happy to have surgeries "without a cut." MIS surgeons often had a lot less convincing to do than he did.

This surgeon explained that there is a large surgical literature describing MIS surgical techniques going back decades. Almost every spine operation imaginable up to and including scoliosis surgery has been reported using MIS technique. However, there isn't a great deal of head-to-head research comparing MIS to more classical "open" surgical technique. And that literature is interesting to consider. Very consistently it says that the benefits of MIS are minor and some complications might actually be more common than they are with old-fashioned "knife-and-fork" surgery.

The surgeon offered to go in and repair the spinal fluid leak but he'd have to do it with an old-fashioned cut, an open exposure. Morris tried to raise his head off the ER stretcher and couldn't because his headache was so bad. *Where do I sign?*

Morris was in the operating room a few hours later. When the surgeon reopened the wound, there was an immediate big gush of warm fluid from it; the new-kid scrub nurse almost passed out! He spread the flesh to expose a large cavity with a smooth silver-gray lining. With fluid leaks internally, the body seemingly attempts to "wall the fluid off" by forming a reactive membrane around it, very similar to the shiny synovial membranes that line our major joints.

The surgeon was able to scrape all that stuff away, and at the bottom of the cavity there was a pinhole communicating down into the spinal canal.

Most of the anatomy he was looking at was intact but the dural sac was tense and tight. He couldn't move it around much with his surgical dissecting tools and that was unusual. It suggested that something was holding the nerve sac in place — maybe a disc hernia? There was very little scarring in the muscle from the MIS procedure five weeks earlier. So where had all that spinal fluid come from? He did a careful exploration of the spinal canal to figure it out, and after some gentle poking and prodding, he found the answer.

After identifying the main nerve sac he retracted it towards the centerline of the body to get to the disc under it and exposed a big soft disc hernia. Lateral to that was the nerve root itself, which looked OK initially.

Our reoperating surgeon made a single "stab wound" incision into the disc bulge with a small scalpel, then reached in with fine surgical graspers called *pituitaries*, which are just 2 or 3 millimeters wide, sometimes smaller. With them he pulled out a great big piece of disc hernia, then a few smaller bits around it. As he did that, the tension came off the main nerve sac and a gush of clear watery spinal fluid flooded the field. *Shit.* He thought he'd torn the main sac in lifting out the hernia.

But he hadn't. After suctioning out the fluid he could confirm the midline sac was intact and the fluid was coming from the undersurface of the nerve root itself. When he lifted the nerve root a bit with his dissectors, he found a crescent-shaped hole in the underside of it, exactly the same shape as the common Kerrison surgical biting tool that we use to trim bone and disc fragments from the surrounding neurological stuff. Fluid was leaking out of it, and there was a thin white stringy bit of stuff hanging out too — the nerve root itself! When he lifted his dissectors away, the nerve root fell back against the disc below it with sufficient pressure to stop the fluid from leaking, at least in the operating room. With Morris lying on his belly in the OR, the spinal fluid pressure was low. But later, when he stood up, gravity would raise the fluid pressure in his low back and a hole like this could leak internally, as it so obviously had.

Putting it all together, it was apparent that the MIS surgeon squinting through the six-inch depth of his access tube had confused the nerve root with the actual disc hernia. When he grabbed the soft bulgy thing that he described as a disc hernia, he was actually grabbing the nerve root, biting off a piece of the surrounding dural sac to cause the spinal fluid leak and tearing out part of the nerve root to cause the numbing drop foot.

The reoperating surgeon was able to patch the hole with special synthetic surgical membrane materials. But you can't repair a torn nerve root, so Morris's neurological deficit would be permanent. He woke up without a headache and by the next morning didn't need the shades. But his foot and leg didn't change. Thankfully the expensive plastic AFO he eventually bought stopped his stumbling and let him return to the office with dignity.

Morris did in fact get voted onto the hospital board, where he tried to drive an initiative to review surgeon outcomes and complications at the boardroom table. Plunking his drop foot splint up onto the table gave him great emphasis and gravitas. But he quickly learned that legally the surgeons were considered "independent contractors" to the hospital; the hospital had no obligation to review their outcomes and was not responsible for them. So he lost his first "case" at the boardroom table!

SPINE CRIMES

Promoting MIS as perfectly safe is another spine crime. It's still surgery, folks, and we can *always* hurt you. Big cut or small.

Chapter 18
Maria's Story

A failing senior failed by many doctors.

People can become quite frail in their old age. They lose their energy and mobility often to the point where they can't live on their own. When their symptoms are all related to mobility, spine surgeons call it *claudication*, and when we use that term, it likely means they're not just getting old.

Maria was lonely. And angry. And frustrated. But beyond it all was a happy disposition that could power a 90-pound 80-year-old matriarch through anything.

The house was very big and very empty after Francesco's passing 10 years before, but she saw reminders of him everywhere she looked, and backache or not she wasn't going anywhere. All three of her children had invited her to live with them, and a decade ago she might have been helpful with the little ones, maybe not running around after them or with homework but with the cooking and the cleaning and just minding the house sometimes. But she couldn't bring herself to leave the house that she and Frank had made a home and where they had made so many memories. Instead, she vowed to keep up the family tradition of Sunday dinner at her big house where they could all be together under one roof.

The weekly ritual kept her busy and gave her life. It was something to look forward to and plan and prepare for. What to serve, what ingredients to shop for, where to get the best of everything. Thank God she could still drive a bit; otherwise how would she get the groceries? And cleaning, sure the children paid for the cleaning service to come in every Friday but Maria didn't want embarrassment. She had to do the place herself on Thursday so it would look OK for strangers from the cleaning company. And then those strangers never did a good-enough job so she'd be cleaning again after they left because if her children saw that her house wasn't perfect, they might try to push her to the nursing home.

The backache didn't help. She'd had it on and off for a long time, mostly when she'd been standing or walking a bit. That was easy to cope with; she'd take a break or do shorter walks. Gradually over the years she'd given up walking to do her errands and now took the car instead. Sometimes on a nice summer day she'd go out for a short stroll but really it was little pleasure to be on her feet. She'd go bench to bench to rest her aching back. She did talk to her doctor about it from time to time. Try this pill or that pill, but they all bothered Maria's stomach so she didn't stick with them and physiotherapy was expensive on a fixed income, so no. In the house she could lean forward to support herself on the mop or the Swiffer or the vacuum and that helped. In the kitchen, she learned to lean forward onto the countertop — that helped a bit too.

She could make her own small meals easily enough but the big weekend cooking became difficult. She'd work at it for 10 or 15 minutes, then take a break to rest her back. Sometimes she would really, really hurt but La Famiglia was coming so she accepted the sacrifice.

Twice in recent months the backache had been so bad Maria had driven herself to the local emergency room to get checked out. The doctor was young enough to be her grandchild but the first ER experience was attentive. A nurse talked nicely to her about the problem for a few minutes and then presented her case to the doctor — she could see them talking down the hall. The doctor then ordered blood tests and low back X-rays. The results were OK except for some arthritis in her low back and he prescribed some arthritis medicine. She took it for a month and added a sore tummy to her list of ailments, but the backache remained. A few weeks after that on a really bad pain day, she went back and saw another doctor who was sympathetic and ordered a CT scan after having the nurse give her a shot of some powerful IV pain medicine. That medicine worked and the scan showed nothing more than the X-rays so with a prescription for the oral form of that IV medicine home she went again. It was Tora-something-or-other and she could take it up to four times a day. It worked and didn't bother her tummy so she got renewals from her family doctor whenever the bottle ran out.

DECOMPENSATION

Toradol worked well but the relief didn't last very long, so Maria still had trouble with the big weekend meal prep. Cooking in 10-minute efforts was awkward, but if she stood for much longer, her legs would start to shake and she just had to sit. Mashing potatoes was the worst, never easy for a small lady, and so she'd save it for the last job after everything else was done and out on the serving platters. She'd mash for a minute, lean forward on the counter to rest, mash another minute.

One Sunday the doorbell rang as she was halfway through her mash. *OMG the kids were early!* They would let themselves in but dinner had to be ready and set out on the table, *had to be*, so she kept mashing as quickly as she could, backache or no . . . and her legs went all rubbery under her. She tried to hold herself up on the kitchen counter but didn't have the strength, and down she slid into a little pile on the floor. She couldn't get up. Her legs wouldn't move.

Mama! Maria found herself surrounded by helping hands and jabbering voices and was hauled up onto her feet and plunked down on a chair at the kitchen table. Her back pain eased and the strength came back to her legs. *No, this had never happened before. No, there was no need to go to the hospital, because what about all this dinner?*

Dinner was great food but lousy conversation, all anybody wanted to talk about was her. She was *embarrassed*! Finding out about jobs and schools and her younger son's new house purchase was like pulling teeth. No, the girls would do the dishes while the boys took her to the ER.

RECEPTION AND "CARE"

At the emergency room a nurse met with Maria and the family and wrote down her story before going off to talk with the doctor. Then the doctor vanished, and everybody sat and waited almost an hour and a half before he reappeared. In a small examining room, he prodded at Maria's back a bit and asked her to move her legs around. He tapped at her knees and ankles with a small rubber hammer and had her lift her legs up off the stretcher. Yes, she could do that.

After the nurse helped her get dressed, the doctor came and spoke with Maria and the family. He explained that her examination and the recent X-rays and CT scan didn't suggest a pinched nerve or tumor or anything bad. Her sons shouted a chorus — but wait, what X-rays? What CT scan? The jig was up, and Maria had to admit she'd been there before. The doctor interrupted all the babbling and said he would admit her into the hospital on the medicine service for a workup and some pain management, so everybody calmed down.

She was admitted into a quiet room of her own with a comfortable bed and nice nurses to look after her. After getting the kids to promise they'd take the dinner leftovers home and clean the kitchen, she let herself relax and fell into an exhausted sleep, right after a technician stuck a needle in her arm and filled a half dozen little glass tubes with blood.

Next morning the nurses woke her up around eight o'clock because breakfast had arrived and the doctors would be coming by on rounds. Breakfast they called it. She wouldn't feed that to her grandson's dog! But she was hungry so after choking it down she let a young lady help her to get dressed and sit up in the bedside chair. Soon a bunch of doctors in long white coats arrived. There were young people in short white coats too and Maria learned that these were the students. After saying "Good morning," nobody really talked to her and they spoke about somebody called "this patient" for a while. Maria heard words like "nonspecific" and "deconditioning" and "long-term care" and they left. Soon her back hurt again and she tried to get back into bed but couldn't. The nurse had to help her.

After lunch one of the short-coat people came by, a young lady who seemed very concerned. Short coat — Maria remembered this was a student. They spoke for almost an hour as she asked Maria about her symptoms, her life and her past medical history. She explained that the "staff" doctor had prescribed pain medicine to be administered regularly, and with the dose going up a bit after every second day, Maria might need to be in hospital for a few weeks until they got the dose right. Because she was old and drugs could be toxic, they had to be careful. *Weeks?*

Ten days later Maria was no better and so constipated her tummy hurt. The doctors did X-rays for that too, then gave her laxatives. On morning rounds the next day, the new staff doctor, a middle-aged woman who Maria learned was the medical ward director for this week, explained she didn't think Maria's current pain meds would work for her, so she was consulting the pain service and ordering an MRI scan.

Every day for a week she was hauled out of bed and wheel-chaired through the hospital to the pain clinic where various needles were stuck into her back and drugs injected through them. The needles all hurt and the drugs never worked. She learned from the pain doctors that her MRI scan showed arthritis and mildly pinched nerves, so when their injections didn't work, they asked a surgeon to see her. *Caramba, no surgery for me,* she thought.

But she did give in and see a surgeon. Another short-coat fellow, another student. After checking his cellphone and typing on it for a while, he did pretty much the same examination she'd had in the ER the first day in and explained that the arthritically swollen joints in her back were pinching the nerves and that scared her. He explained that this was a common "false positive" finding — a common thing in old people that could cause sciatica, but because she had only back pain there was nothing to be done. This young man had learned that surgeons can't treat back pain, only leg pain or sciatic weakness, and because she didn't have those problems surgery would not be an option for her.

She was happy to hear that but — *what about my pain, Doctor?* Maria learned that the dose of her pain medicines would be increased to try to get her comfortable while she was waiting for a rehab bed, which could take a few weeks. *Why do I need a rehab bed?* That's how we "manage" patients like you. If you do really well there, you might even be able to get back home . . .

Manage? Oh crap, these doctors don't want to let me go home. Maria grabbed the phone as soon as that doctor left and called her kids in a panic. She wanted out. The kids came in and there was a long conference with the staff doctor where it was confirmed to the family that the patient couldn't be discharged. She was so weak she'd be falling and was unsafe. Maybe she could eventually be released with a wheelchair, once she adjusted to it.

Hospital assimilation complete. Maria wasn't Maria anymore. She was reduced to being The Patient who had failed all treatments.

Three days later The Patient's pain was better but she was very very sleepy all the time. One morning the team of doctors woke her up on morning rounds. That made her mad. The staff doctor (*What is that anyway?*) explained that she couldn't continue on the dose of drugs she needed for the pain because they were too strong (which was why she was sleeping all the time) and that had complications. So, he was going to ask another surgeon . . . *Zzzzzzzzzzzzzzzzzzzzz* . . . Maria, Maria, wake up . . . for a second opinion about her back.

REDEMPTION AND RESCUE

Later that afternoon a man came by her bedside, no lab coat but a shirt and tie and a hospital ID badge. As he shook her awake, Maria could see that his jeans were scruffy and his thinning gray hair all messed up. *What kind of doctor was this?* He apologized for waking her up and started to explain . . . *Zzzzzzzzzzzzzzzzzzzzzzzzz.*

Next morning Maria's back was sore, and when she asked for pain medicine, she didn't get any. The nurse explained that the doctor had ordered her pain medicine to be stopped for some kind of a test. He'd written that she could have some Tylenol, which she gladly took, and it helped a little bit.

Early that evening, after dinner, the fellow with the scruffy jeans showed up again. When he admitted that, yes, he was the one who had stopped her pain medicines, Maria lit into him in Italian and he almost had to shout to calm her down.

This doctor was different; he sat down in the bedside chair and talked to her about her back pain, asking a number of simple questions. Not about her life or her illnesses or whether the medicines or injections had worked but about her pain.

When did it start?

About 10 years ago, maybe six months after her Francesco passed away. She and Francesco used to walk together for almost an hour every day, outside when the weather was good and in the mall when it wasn't.

How did she first notice it?

She had kept up with her long walks, but they were lonely without Francesco. And then she started feeling very tired and sore at the end of each walk.

What would she do about it?

Nothing. She just walked less and less. Sometimes she'd stop and sit on a bench for a rest. Two years ago she'd given up on her walks entirely and started driving everywhere to do her errands.

Did it move around, go to other parts of her body like her shoulders or her tummy or her bum or her legs?

Not really, but sometimes just before her legs got rubbery, it would spread to her hips a bit.

Then the doctor asked her if she knew where her hips were and could she point to them. *Idiot doctor! Everybody knows where the hip is*, she thought, pointing at her buttocks! He grinned a bit.

If it hurt too much to walk, what would she do to get relief?

In the mall could she just stop and window shop a bit? No, she had to sit down or bend forward. Sometimes she leaned on the shopping cart all the way through the grocery store.

He grinned some more, then he asked her to stand up and walk a few steps in the room for him. *Why? Nobody else had ever asked her to do that.* Apparently he wanted to check for any limp. Maria was too weak to get out of bed by this point, so the doctor actually got up and helped her. *Wow, he really was different!* She hauled herself all the way up to her five-foot-two height, but couldn't stand straight for more than a second or two. It just hurt too much to try to look the doctor in the eye and so she sagged forward onto her walker. To walk she'd heave the walker forward a foot or so, then drag her legs after it. Not great. When the doctor tried to take the walker away, she hung onto it for dear life, so he gently led her back to the bed.

With her lying down, he asked her to push against the strength of his hands with all the various muscles of her leg, and she was strong! He tapped her knees and ankles with a rubber hammer thing and nothing happened when he did. He tested her ability to feel him touch her legs and feet at several points, and she could feel all of that. He played with her big toe, moving it up and down, and asked her to say whether it was up or down without looking, and she could do that.

Then he sat back down in the bedside chair and talked. He explained that the swollen joints of arthritis in her back were just like bunions, that there was one on either side of the middle of her back and that those swellings were pinching the nerves — that's called *spinal stenosis*. It commonly causes not everyday, all-the-time backache but something called *claudication*, symptoms that get worse with standing up straight or walking and are relieved by rest and bending forward, which unpinches the nerves a bit. Those symptoms are highly variable — back pain, numbness and tingling in the legs, weakness, limp, sometimes in different combinations.

This doctor offered her a surgery. It would be a small operation but no surgery in an 80-year-old was to be taken lightly. He'd want a bunch of heart tests and a cardiology consult beforehand, and she might have to go into ICU for a while afterwards. But with her symptoms and anatomy, there was an excellent chance she'd be much better off after surgery — not perfect, but much better able to stand and walk and live a normal daily life. She'd likely be able to stay in her home and not need the long-term rehab bed she was now on a wait list for.

Surgery! Could she die? Yes. *Could she be paralyzed?* Yes.

What if she didn't have it? She'd stay as she was, in pain and unable to walk much and needing an assisted living facility. And she would slowly get worse, as she had already been doing for 10 years.

Maybe. But first, Dottore, you check my heart and talk with my family.

The next three days were a blur of tests and consults with cardiology and anesthesiology. At dinnertime her three children and their partners came to the hospital and the doctor showed up. He explained the claudication thing and that Maria's nerves were pinched not just at one disc level but two. He would operate on both in one procedure. It was a small thing, commonly a day surgery in people who were younger and healthy and not so badly off. The actual surgery would take about an hour and a half. The

ICU was simply a precaution. He didn't really expect there would be a need, and the cardiology testing had been excellent.

There was a lot of talking. The doctor excused himself to go see his other inpatients and came back 45 minutes later to learn the decision was *Yes!*

Two days later Maria spent three hours in an operating room, roughly half and half anesthesia time and surgery. She lost about 100cc or four ounces of blood. She woke up only a bit sore and didn't need much more than Tylenol — certainly she didn't need an ICU bed.

The next day she could stand straighter for longer and more comfortably than she had in years, but her legs were still shaky. *Why, Doctor?* Madam, remember those legs haven't worked much or been exercised for years, so they won't be perfect overnight! Research suggests that measurable gains in strength might be going on for a year and a half. Oh yes, he'd said that beforehand.

A few days later the hospital staff said she should be transferred to inpatient rehab because she was so rubbery and weak to begin with. Less than two weeks later she decided she wanted to go home and another family conference was called. Her kids made up a schedule where somebody could stay with her every day for the first few weeks, and home she went.

A month later she was walking well with a cane, not using it in the house, and feeling so good that she could stand long enough to make a good meal again. She even brought a fresh-baked lasagna to the doctor's office at her follow-up appointment. No pain. Good lasagna!

Maria didn't show up for her two-month visit so the doctor had his nurse call up to check on her. She apologized for missing her appointment and explained that she was too busy. There was a big bake sale on for the church and she was engaged with that, and she had spent enough time with doctors already.

The surgeon told his nurse to wish the patient well and welcome her back anytime.

How is it that Maria was denied care the first time around and left to get worse and worse? This spine crime happens regularly around the world and can easily lead to terrible, even tragic, outcomes.

Many if not most doctors get very little spine care education and back pain is a particularly deep dark black hole of ignorance. Even in the medical community, the belief (nay, misunderstanding) is that people never get better, backache always comes back and surgery has no role.

The misconception that "surgery doesn't work" goes back to the very beginnings of spine care. Two fundamental articles were published out of Boston way back in 1911 reporting that fusion surgery could relieve back pain. The concept took off like a rocket, but whereas fusion works well for painfully arthritic joints in the arms and legs, it's a bust for "nonspecific" back pain associated with worn-out discs. That's been proven time and time again in scientific literature going back over a century.

Notice I didn't say "it doesn't work" here, I said, "It's a bust for 'nonspecific' back pain associated with worn-out discs," and that's true. Surgery works well for two generic things other than neurological compressions: instability and deformity. Those two 1911 articles? One was about a series of untreated scoliosis cases (deformity) and one was largely on a series of patients whose spines had been rotted away by tuberculosis infection (instability).

Spinal stenosis is not one simple thing. There are many anatomical variants of stenosis and it can be associated with instability and deformity, so getting the *complete* diagnosis right can be tricky. The surgery can get complicated but bottom line, when it's appropriate for a specific case and done right, it works well.

The key symptom in spinal stenosis isn't backache or sciatic pain or numbness or tingling or weakness in the legs, any or all of which may or may not be present. It's claudication: the fact that whatever symptoms are bothering the patient get worse when the patient is standing erect and/or walking around and are relieved only when the patient bends forward (because that position enlarges the spinal canal and unpinches the nerves a bit). Too many practitioners forget that.

Maria was almost prematurely doomed to a life of chronic pain and immobility in a nursing home because that first "surgeon" consultant (a student really, his staff supervisor never saw Maria — that's another issue we could talk about) didn't know much more than what his teachers had taught him: *You can't treat back pain with surgery.*

A great deal of surgical training today focuses on acquiring procedural skills without delivering a good understanding of which procedure is best done when. That student was also too busy or couldn't be bothered to take a proper history of Maria's symptoms. Later the consultant surgeon who did offer her surgery found that just a short bedside conversation proved to be enough to pick up the claudication issue.

Neuro-claudication — back, buttock and/or leg symptoms increased with erect posture or walking, which are relieved by flexion rest — is the salient symptom of lumbar spinal stenosis. Not pain. Not weakness. Not numbness or tingles. Sadly, too many doctors and surgeons are unaware of the unique cluster of symptoms that constitute claudication and are, therefore, unable to make an accurate diagnosis.

Heads up, there's another syndrome, vascular claudication, caused by the hardening of the arteries. Worse with activity; better with rest. But it's different in many obvious ways — no sciatic pain, no relief with bending forward, leg symptoms almost exclusively in the shin and top of the foot, and associated with cold feet or dark discoloration of the toes. FYI.

To be fair, lots of spinal stenosis is without symptoms, maybe most of it. If your scan shows some pinched nerves, don't get all excited. Without symptoms, nothing needs to be done. But if you've had claudication symptoms regularly for more than six months or so, they likely won't be going away, and those symptoms do tend to progress over time.

How quickly will things deteriorate? That's highly variable, but in an individual case it seems the patient can look forward in time by looking back. If a few months ago things weren't much different than they are now, then a few months later things won't likely be much different either, so we can all watch and wait. However, if a few months ago you were fine and month to month your symptoms are getting worse, then it may be time to book some surgery.

If your stenosis symptoms are just pain and you have good mobility, we have lots of treatment that can help short of surgery. Drugs, physical medicine treatments, injections, rehab, you name it. Often some simple modifications of lifestyle and activity make a big difference, as they do for my own very chronic back pain. These things never cure all the pain but they manage it and can make it quite tolerable.

If you're having trouble standing and walking and your legs are getting weak, it may be decision time. If bone spurs are crushing your nerves, ultimately somebody has to cut those spurs away. When? Simple. When you have symptoms *that you can't live with*. Spine surgery is very much quality-of-life surgery, and that makes it a very subjective decision. Some people may go undiagnosed or delay things for too long. People like Maria who can barely stand and walk should have it dealt with ASAP. If you're not so badly off, decide if you can live with it or not.

The real spine crime? Surgeons who don't know anything other than surgery, who never really learn to talk to a patient. That's too many of us.

Chapter 19
Jack's Back-Breaking Job

Not just another compensation client trying to game the system.

Jack was the back pain case no surgeon wants to see and too many doctors love to treat. We know that neurological spine syndromes, deformity and instability are the only three things that can respond well to surgical care, but backache, what we professionally call back-dominant pain, not so much. On day one, most of us assume this guy's never going to get better and so, if insured, he can generate billing activity for us for years.

Jack had done hard physical work in the mills all his short life. Back-breaking work, as it turns out. Backache started in his late 20s, narcotics in his 30s, and by his 40s he had been on workers' compensation with back pain a half dozen times. He'd been treated and rehabbed up the wazoo, always "doing well" but always hurting himself again on the job very quickly. He never hurt his back at home or playing golf or going fishing, curiously always at work. The ER knew him well, his X-rays always looked the same (they showed *all* his discs were badly worn out), his pain was always terrible and a prescription for Percocet was always sent home with him.

One day he didn't go straight home from the ER. His pain was so bad, even after he was given several Percs to take. They hooked up an IV and gave him some morphine; that helped. But you can't send a guy dependent on IV drugs home, can you? So the spine service was consulted, and in the middle of the night he was admitted. An MRI scan was scheduled for the next morning.

Shocking surprise, like the X-rays, the MRI scan showed that every single one of the discs in his low back was badly worn out. No big hernias and no stenosis reported, reasonable alignment too. The report said "diffuse disc degeneration . . . no change from multiple previous . . . nonsurgical."

In hospital, the pain service was consulted. They adjusted his meds daily and gave him a mix of drugs, some of which were long-acting and some short-acting. They worked better than the Percs, and with pain eased off a bit, Jack was able to get up and hobble around enough to get home. After a few weeks he was down to his usual stiff and sore, and with bills to pay it was time to work again. But both his employer and the compensation board said no. He'd have to have a physical assessment test of some sort by one of their people and likely do some rehab for at least a month or two before he would be safe to return to work.

The testing wasn't very impressive. After waiting around for almost an hour after his appointment was supposed to begin, he was ushered into an exam room by a bored-looking fellow in a lab coat who asked him a few questions about his pain and then did a quick physical exam. It took all of three minutes and consisted of asking him to touch his toes and bend backwards, and tapping his knee and ankle reflexes with a hammer.

Could Jack touch his toes? *Never was much of an athlete, never could.* Try, said his assessor.

OK. Deep breath, grunt, suck in the gut and bend. Not bad, it didn't hurt and his fingertips made it almost all the way down to his ankles before that gut got in the way. But then he almost got stuck, trying to come back up hurt like hell. He had to bend his knees a bit and put his hands on his thighs and then bit by bit he could inch his hands up his thighs to get straight without too much pain. Then he had to bend backwards; that was better.

Fantastic, he was told. He was sooo flexible! He didn't need *any* rehab with that kind of mobility. Stiffness causes a lot of disability and if you can't bend, you can't work. That kind of stiffness can get a guy a 20 percent pension for life from the compensation board, but Jack could bend so much he'd only get 5 percent if he felt he couldn't work. *Who can live on that?*

So Jack returned to work. Things were great for three weeks and then ... *Bam!* He had a huge cramp of pain again, dropped the load he was carrying and hit the ground. Back to the hospital as the boss yelled how Jack was just another compensation jerk and wasn't coming back to his company ever again.

Same deal in the hospital. More meds. This time the pain service guy consulted the addictions service because Jack's drug doses were so high. Great way to connect with a bedridden man in pain, suggest he's faking it all to get high as if he was living La Vida Loca in his hospital bed with the bedside urinal. He wasn't, and he sent the addictions lady away to think about that. Did his best to be polite, didn't throw the urinal at anybody.

This time the meds weren't working and the pain guy suggested they try some cortisone injections into his back. That helped a bit. Three days later a second shot got him out of bed, and three days after that a third got him moving well enough to go home.

A month later when his boss refused to consider taking him back, he made an appointment at compensation again. This time he saw an enthusiastic young doctor who was very concerned and asked him to bend again. Jack wasn't stupid, no more of that for him and so he stopped with his fingertips at the upper thigh just below the groin. The doctor got very serious and told him that was bad. He'd need inpatient rehab at the compensation board hospital.

The rehab place didn't work out well. Therapists took him to the gym every day for three weeks, bend and stretch. You're young; you can do it. He couldn't and eventually they gave up, wrote a report, and Jack got his 20 percent benefit and an early retirement.

Great, just great. Twenty percent of his former salary from compensation and his state income support package gave him just enough to live on after selling the truck and quitting smoking (insurance and cigarettes were expensive). His wife, Jennifer, took a job at the local grocery store to help pay the bills.

But he still hurt despite all the meds he continued to take.

As time wore on, Jack got increasingly desperate with his pain. The slightest movement hurt; he could barely wash and even toileting was a problem. What a life. He thought very seriously about ending it. Why not? Just close the garage door one day while Jen was at work and turn on the car. He badgered his family doctor for a referral to a doctor outside the compensation system. It might help, and workers' compensation would still cover it.

He was indeed referred to a surgeon, but this was yet another doctor at the compensation offices. He asked him a few questions about his back but he seemed to be more interested in Jack's legs, which were now constantly aching too. He poked and prodded at his back a bit, tested the strength of his leg muscles and did the reflexes thing again. Nope, nothing to do, this was just back-dominant pain, and surgery apparently can't help that.

Jack wasn't happy, wasn't impressed. Frustrated and back at his family doctor's office, he asked for yet another referral, for a second surgical opinion. This surgeon was different. After having new X-rays done standing up, Jack was interrogated aggressively about the details of his pain and the flareups, about his walking and bending and what he could or couldn't do at home.

The surgeon gently felt along all his back, butt and hip muscles, asked him to bend and twist his body in a few different directions, let him back off when bending forward started to hurt, and Jack thought she smiled a bit when he put his hands on his thighs to come back up again.

When done with her examination, she left Jack to look at the scans and X-rays. When she came back she reassured him that there were no disc bulges or pinched nerves in his back; nothing was going to paralyze him.

Duh, this has been going on for more than 20 years and I'm not paralyzed yet!

She explained that the discs in the spine act like bearings, guiding the motion between our vertebrae, and that every single one of Jack's discs was shot. He was getting those odd, sudden flareups of his pain because he was periodically "jamming" or going out of joint just a little bit. This was a rare problem called *internal lumbar disc derangement* (ILDD), meaning that the disc was injured within itself rather than being ruptured or pushed out of place. Doc explained that ILDD is typically diagnosed in a younger spine and commonly has people standing all kinds of crooked as their body seeks a position to offload the injury (*Oh yeah, that's me . . .*) and that it usually takes at least several days, sometimes weeks or even months for things to jiggle back into place so the pain might settle down and the patient can stand up straight again.

So, Doc, there's nothing that can be done about it, right? With the bearings all shot we scrap the car? Maybe not. Come to the consult office; let's look at your MRI together.

WTF, look at my MRI? Nobody had had Jack do that before. The surgeon pointed out the bones and discs and neurological stuff, showed how the nerves weren't pinched and the discs weren't bulging. Then she pointed at one, second from the bottom (L4/L5) and said, "Look at the bone marrow around it." Compared to the other discs, the bone marrow here was finely discoloured. The surgeon explained that this was likely a reflection of inflammation in that disc, suggesting it was more a source of pain than the others. Not hard proof, but a strong hint. *Makes sense.*

Then the surgeon put up the new standing X-rays and showed Jack how his spine collapsed through his L4/L5 disc when he stood up. There was a little scoliosis tilt there, looking at things from the front. Looking from the side, the L4 bone had slipped forward on L5 below it by a few millimeters — not much, not hard proof, but all very suggestive of mechanical trouble there. *Makes sense.*

If Jack couldn't live with his current level of chronic pain, a stabilizing operation at that L4/L5 level might help. The intention was not to make him perfect or pain free (with all his discs being worn, that was never going to happen) but to stop the flareups and *ease* his pain a great deal.

What are the odds, Doc? She explained that, historically, fusion for back pain from a disc helps about 70 percent of people to be better off — never perfect, but better. With the clinical ILDD diagnosis and strong hints in the imaging that L4/L5 was the culprit disc, the surgeon said she'd be very surprised if Jack wouldn't be better off. She added that interbody bone grafts and cage implants were commonly used to fix this problem, with 85 to 90 percent success rates reported in the original research literature. *Not bad.* This ILDD thing was a rare problem. The surgeon treated a case maybe every two or three months and only once every two or three years somebody went through it all and didn't get better — do the arithmetic.

Jack asked, *How long until I'll need another fusion surgery?* Several guys at the mill had had the same operation and nobody ever seemed to get more than a few years out of them.

Good question. The surgeon explained that in a badly worn-out spine, there was a 3 percent chance per year of life that something else would go wrong and need more work after fusion surgery. *Wow!*

The surgeon went back to Jack's standing X-rays and did a bunch of angle measurements on the computer screen. Then she smiled a bit, said that actually Jack's spine had a significant degenerative deformity and that there was a trend in very recent research data suggesting that the need for reoperation was very much lessened if fusion was done in such a way as to get the alignment right, and that was something that could likely be achieved with surgery for Jack.

Better and better! Where do I sign?

The fusion surgery went well. Jack stayed in the hospital overnight and went home the next morning, sore as hell from the cut and needing his meds (and more!) for that, but with the old original pain feeling better right off.

The pain of the cut started to ease around three weeks and Jack started weaning off his meds. At two months he was using less than he had been before surgery, X-rays looked good and the surgeon started him exercising to get his strength back.

Long story short, six months later Jack was taking just two extra-strength Tylenol tablets daily, one each at breakfast and lunch because he woke up very stiff. He could bend enough to tie his own shoes, and he could play with his young grandkids in ways he never had.

Jack never did go back to the mill. But he did take a job at the local Chevy dealer, shuttling customers around, which put a little money in his pocket, got him out of the house and gave Jen some peace. She liked it at the grocer's so she kept at it.

SPINE CRIMES

Jack was no jerk trying to game the compensation system. He was a victim of it. We might want to say that all those doctors and paramedicals who treated him so unsuccessfully through all the years of his getting worse and worse were jerks, but they weren't really; in the majority, they're just ignorant. Not stupid or uncaring but not well educated in all the not-so-little things (like kinetics and biomechanics, among other subjects) that can really help a doctor to understand a spine care patient. Spine is not a major thing in the general medical curriculum. But clearly it should be.

Telling the patient with "just" back pain and no other symptoms, the back-dominant spine patient, that there's no hope is another common spine crime. Even if the odds of good outcome are just 70 percent, that's not a bad gamble for a world of people in often desperate circumstance who have tried all the nonsurgical care options unsuccessfully. In fact, those odds are way better than nothing and way better than accepting a life of pain and misery. A 70 percent chance of major improvement in quality of life shouldn't be denied to anybody.

Chapter 20
Theo Didn't Get Better

Right surgery, wrong disc.

Theo was in the prime of life, a 54-year-old restaurateur whose thriving business let him support his family in style. Big house, great cars, a fine family vacation every summer. Louisa had everything she ever wanted. The kids had gone to the best schools and universities thanks to Dad's largesse, graduating with no debt. The first grandchild was on the way.

You work hard in the restaurant business. You get tired, you get sore. That happened a lot to Theo, but he was a hustler and accepted that as the price of success. Tylenol was his friend.

Late one summer when his backache started to flare after a holiday, the Tylenol didn't work and after a few weeks of increasing agony Theo found time to stop by his doctor's office. The doctor examined him, found nothing and, after checking that his patient's blood pressure was OK, suggested that Theo switch to Advil, which might be more effective in alleviating his back pain. Advil and other anti-inflammatory drugs like it can affect the kidneys, causing fluid retention and elevating the blood pressure, so Theo would have to monitor that.

Theo was a big guy, so he took the maximum dose of Advil (400 mg tablets three times a day) religiously for three weeks, but they didn't work. Maybe a bit at first but the pain was back in the second week and worse by the third, so he went back to the doctor. He was really feeling stiff and sore all over now. After examining him a second time, again with normal results, his GP sighed and said he should try some physio, and let's get an X-ray just in case. *OK, fine.*

Two days later the phone rang at the restaurant. The doctor told Theo there was a lot of arthritis in his X-ray, and because of his worsening pain the doctor wanted him to get an MRI scan done as soon as possible. *OK, fine.*

Squeezing himself onto the narrow scanning table was tough and his back and legs hurt lying down on that hard surface, so they had to get him a bunch of pillows to prop up his knees and shoulders before he could stay still long enough to do it.

Monday afternoon the phone rang at the restaurant again and the doctor wanted to see him right away. *Could I come first thing tomorrow morning? We're busy right now.* The doctor was not happy about waiting, but OK.

Theo didn't sleep that night. Neither did Louisa.

Next morning the doctor looked really serious and explained that the arthritis in Theo's spine had caused bone spurs to grow and those spurs were pinching his spinal cord a bit below his shoulder blades. In a big way. The scan report said the spinal cord was "highly compressed." Theo should see a surgeon as soon as possible. *Yessir!*

Later that week, Theo and Louisa met the surgeon at his downtown office across the street from the hospital. He spent a good half hour interviewing Theo about all his symptoms and examining him thoroughly, had him stand and walk and even take a short jog, bend all around, stand on one foot and the other. Theo was proud: he could do it all despite his pain — but he was so sore that even when the surgeon tapped his knee and ankle reflexes, the jump of Theo's legs hurt.

The surgeon frowned a lot. After the examination he left the room "for a look at the scan," and when he returned he asked Theo and Louisa to come to his consult suite to see the scan for themselves. The surgeon pointed out what was front and back in the scan picture, what was disc and what was spine bone, and where the spinal cord was a gray streak of flesh floating in the middle of a white bath of spinal fluid. Then he magnified one part of the scan and even Theo could see that the gray streak of flesh was pinched badly by some black stuff behind it, and the white spinal fluid bath was nowhere to be seen there.

The surgeon explained that the black stuff was arthritic bone spurring opposite the T9/T10 disc and it was damaging Theo's spinal cord already. That's why his legs were so achy and jumpy with the reflex test. He said he was surprised that Theo wasn't worse off and explained that once a compressed spinal cord was symptomatic, it pretty much never got better by itself and tended over time to do nothing but get worse. Maybe it was a good idea to get those spurs out.

The surgeon explained that this was a common smaller spine operation; Theo would need two laminectomies done at T9 and T10 to allow for safe removal of all those spurs. It wasn't quite a day case, but for the insurance they could make it look like a day case by keeping Theo in hospital overnight and discharging him home at 23 hours. Of course if there were problems or if Theo was too sore to go home, he could be kept in.

Problems? What problems? Give me the good and the bad, Doc.

The surgeon explained that with successful surgery not only would Theo stop getting worse, there was likely a 90 percent chance his spinal cord symptoms would slowly get somewhat better as his spinal cord healed over the course of a year. (*What, not perfectly better?* Nope, it was too late for that.) There was a small chance he might not get better at all but that wasn't expected in his case. Because his neurological symptoms were minor and he was in relatively good shape coming to surgery, he'd likely do well. Common risks were death, infection, blood clots, paralysis and "mechanical" problems at the surgery site that might need reoperation with screws. (*Death? Paralysis? Screws?*)

Theo hugged Louisa and thought about crying a bit but didn't. *How soon could it happen?* Next week. *No, can we look at the week after that? I need some time.* OK, and Theo signed the papers.

When they got home, Theo and Louisa cried a lot. Next day he called the priest and got a special blessing. Then he called his lawyer and his accountant and they all met a few times to get the papers in order just in case something went wrong. Theo didn't have much life insurance but the business was doing very well and needed protecting for the family.

THE SURGERY

Theo's surgery was scheduled in the morning. He came to in the recovery room afterwards with bright lights and beeping machines all around him as voices mumbled at the bedside. The OR team was handing over to the recovery room team but nobody gave him any specifics.

There were IVs in both arms and a catheter Down There and what felt like a lump between his shoulder blades — that was the dressing over the swollen surgical wound. And pain, but not much pain. Mostly a deep dull ache, not much more intense than the pre-op pain. Theo could move his arms and wiggle on the stretcher quite comfortably. When he moved his left arm, he bumped up against a round plastic thing about six inches across with a long bloody really big IV tube sticking out of it. The nurse said that was a suction drain drawing blood out of the wound so he wouldn't get a hematoma there.

Hmm. The pre-op pain. Still there. That's odd. Was it odd? Who knew? This was a new experience for Theo ... but hadn't his surgeon said it was a 9/10 probability that he'd wake up with the old pain gone? And he still felt it. OK so Theo was one in 10; he could live with that and the pain was more than bearable with all these caring nurses asking how sore he was and slipping wonder drugs into his IV if he said he was sore at all.

After a while, his surgeon came by and asked him how he felt. Yup, he was the one in 10. The surgeon told Theo that his spinal cord had been awfully squished; it really was a wonder that he wasn't worse off. He examined the strength and feeling in his legs a bit, much the same way the nurses already had done 10 or 15 times, and pronounced Theo "OK."

Getting out of the car at home was tough because Theo had stiffened up a lot, and his legs were still rubbery. *Why are they still rubbery?* Louisa reminded Theo that the doctor had said it sometimes takes a few weeks before the nerves start to work better.

AFTERMATH

Two weeks later at the doctor's office, the stitches came out of a well-healed wound that didn't hurt at all. The old back pain was still there, though, and the legs were still rubbery. The surgeon said it was too early to send Theo for physio; he wanted the wound to heal for a few more weeks, but he didn't want Theo to be a couch potato either so he asked his patient to take a brisk walk at least once if not twice a day and booked physio to start in three more weeks.

The walking wasn't easy; Theo's legs were still rubbery and stiff like before.

The physio was interesting, lots of stretching everywhere and some leg strengthening. Three times a week for six weeks. Theo and Louisa kept up the walking too, but it wasn't easy because his legs were still not working well. He wobbled a lot and really liked to lean on Louisa's arm to steady himself. He was a big man and Louisa was a small lady. One day when he stumbled and he saw her wince as she supported his weight, he decided to get a cane.

At three months after surgery, neither Theo nor the surgeon was happy. The surgeon said he certainly would expect a patient to be somewhat better at three months. Maybe something else was going on? The surgeon suggested Theo get nerve testing done on his legs.

Because of his diabetes and high blood pressure he might have something called *neuropathy*, a degenerative disease of the nerves themselves that can slow or even stop healing from happening. *That made sense.*

The tests confirmed: "mild to moderate sensorimotor peripheral neuropathy." Unfortunately, there's no real treatment for neuropathy. It's "managed" by making sure the treatable causes of it are looked after, and so Theo had a bunch of tests looking at his diabetes control, circulation, thyroid and B12 levels, which were all fine. If leg pains from it were an issue, there were special meds to deal with that, but Theo's pain was all in his back. The surgeon said there was still hope for benefit from the surgery. The scientific literature suggested that operated spinal cords can improve progressively for a year.

At a year Theo was so unsteady he needed a walker even inside the house and couldn't really go out at all. The surgeon said, "It is what it is." There was simply nothing more he could do for Theo.

RESOLUTION

A year later Theo needed the walker all the time and hadn't been able to get back into the restaurant at all. Louisa had struggled to run it with some help from the kids, but it didn't work out so he'd sold it and had to lay everybody off. His back pain had remained an issue and one day when he was at his family doctor's office getting prescription refills, he asked about getting another scan, maybe another surgeon's opinion. The fellow who had looked after him was a very nice guy with all kinds of certificates on his walls but who knows? His doctor waffled and admitted he didn't want to anger a surgeon by referring a case that had already been treated, but he agreed to at least get the scan done. If the report said there was something there, he'd refer.

The scan happened just over a week later, and a few days after that his doctor's office called with an appointment to see another surgeon across town.

This new surgeon wasn't a happy guy. He didn't smile at all. He spent a lot of time with Theo asking about his symptoms before and since the surgery, and then examined him very thoroughly, testing not just his strength but also what he could feel and something called *two-point discrimination* that Theo couldn't feel at all. Really, his feet were quite completely numb now from the ankles down. This surgeon asked Theo to stand and walk around a bit but he couldn't; he fell over without the walker or a wall to lean on. Through all this, there was a lot of frowning. Then he left the exam room "to look over the scan again" and came back to invite Theo and Louisa to see it with him, just as the first surgeon had.

He pointed out some anatomy, including the black spurs squishing the spinal cord and the scar from the surgery at the T8/T9 level. The surgeon pointed out something new too: there was a big white swelling in Theo's spinal cord just above and below the spurs at T9/T10, which the doctor called *myelomalacia*, a sign of scarring in the spinal cord and not a good thing.

Wait a minute. Time slowed down for Theo and his vision blurred and even his hearing went funny as the doctor pointed to those black spurs and explained that they were still there. The scar from surgery was at T8/T9. The spinal cord compression was at T9/T10. Surgery had been done at the wrong level and Theo's spinal cord was still compressed.

Oh shit.

Theo took a few deep breaths, and as he calmed himself, his vision cleared, his hearing settled and he could think again.

There was no denying this mistake. Did Theo want to sue his first surgeon? No, Theo wanted to get better. *Doctor, can you operate? Can you help me out now?*

That frown deepened. Like the first surgeon, this doctor explained that damaged spinal cords have a limited healing potential and the best predictor of how a patient would do is their condition coming into the surgery. Theo was pretty badly off now. He could still improve even with his neuropathy, likely would improve, but he'd almost certainly never stand and walk normally again.

Theo asked if he should have had another scan after the surgery to make sure his spinal cord had been thoroughly decompressed. No, doing that routinely would mean a great deal of unnecessary scanning and cost because this was such a rare situation.

Should I have had another post-surgery scan, done earlier? Doctor, would you have ordered one for me? Frown, mumble. It was like pulling teeth but Theo got him to admit that yes, he would have, likely around the six-month point in a case where the patient wasn't getting better, and maybe earlier than that for a patient who was really badly off. That was *his* usual practice, but there were no rules on the question that he was aware of.

Right, let's operate. Risk/benefit discussion again. Surgeon 2 was worried about scarring in the surgical field and particularly on the dural sac that contained the spinal fluid bathing the spinal cord. It might tear at surgery and repairing it could be a challenge. *This is no life, Doc, go for it.*

When Theo woke up again, it was awesome — that pain between his shoulder blades was finally gone and his legs felt better, not perfect but stronger, right away. And his feet weren't numb. He was better on his feet almost immediately and mobile enough to go home with his walker on the third day.

This time physios from home care came to the house and started his leg strengthening exercises early. They felt good this time!

He started at the outpatient rehab clinic a month later and they wanted to get him walking between the parallel bars but he grinned, held his hands above the bars and walked along unsupported, so they brought out his walker. He aced the walker. They tried two canes and he could do it.

After a couple of months, it was just one cane, and he could "wall-walk" the house to get to the bathroom without it. He took the cane outside and got the mail for the first time in two years. He and Louisa celebrated at what used to be his second-favorite restaurant (his own place had always been best!) and he walked in from the car without the cane, just Louisa supporting him. They cried all through their meal.

A year after the second surgery Theo still needed his cane on long walks but he had no pain and could look after himself in an elementary way, even do some shopping and whatnot. He could pick up and hold his grandson without falling over, and a granddaughter was on the way!

His surgeon said he'd done better than expected and was ready to discharge him. "You've got what you're going to get."

Hmm. Do I need another scan, Doc? Neurologically no, but if you're worried that I might have botched up like the last guy we can order one for reassurance's sake. *No, I'm OK.*

What about suing? Theo, if you want to go after the first surgeon who botched the operation, it has to be done within a certain timeframe. *For what, Doc, I have money and an OK life now thanks to you. It won't make me better, will it?*

Theo, you should sue for your costs, for your future medical care and medicines and rehab and all that … oh yeah, wait a minute, you got better and don't need much of that.

Theo had a parting thought. *Doc, if he can do this to me, maybe he's doing it to other people too and he needs to know to be more careful. Would you speak to him?*

Frown, mumble. Bottom line, no. Surgeon 2 thought that Surgeon 1 would just take that as an attack on his business and not really care. It would be much more powerful coming from Theo himself in the form of a letter to the medical board and copied to the chief of surgery at the hospital.

So Theo and Louisa wrote a letter. And moved on.

SPINE CRIMES

Not thoroughly following up on a case that's not recovering well, or that's getting worse, is a medical crime in general. Hypertension? Prescribe blood pressure medicines, recheck the blood pressure and if it's still high, prescribe more. Diabetes? Check the blood sugar, adjust the insulin dose if it's still too high. And it's no different in spine care. A patient's worsening condition demands thorough examination and testing. Furthermore, in this case, the patient was worse post-surgery. Simply doing nerve conduction tests at that point was garbage; nerve disease bad enough to cause disability is rare compared to spine problems, and it almost never brings a case to the point where they're falling down.

Failed response to spine surgery should be investigated first and foremost for nothing other than persisting or new spine problems (here, that meant the MRI scan that was eventually done). Why? In the majority we can *fix* spine problems. You can't fix neuropathy!

As for doing surgery on the wrong level of the spine, it's really easy to approach the wrong disc level. When we get in there, the posterior bony anatomy that we see first doesn't differ much from one bone to the other, and those discs aren't very far apart. We take X-rays on the way in to try to be sure of things, but those OR images are often very poor quality and hard to interpret. But once we get in there, it's generally obvious when things don't look right. We should take more X-rays and go to the right place if we've missed!

Chapter 21

Ricardo's Wreckage

When good care goes bad.

Ricardo was a great big tall guy, six foot six if an inch and a solid 240 pounds. He was lean and hard and blessed with the sort of metabolism that keeps some lucky people that way well into middle age. Naturally, he did a lot of sports and athletics in his younger years but his interests ranged much wider than that, and after engineering school he went on to a successful business career.

Long hours at a desk can be hard on a guy and sure enough by late middle age Ric had some backache. He went through a few different ergonomic chairs and played with a standing desk and all these things helped him get the job done but once you're sore, you're sore. He'd have trouble standing up straight at the end of the day, and in his late 50s he liked his Tylenol a lot. When that stopped working, he went through chiro and physio, then he had an MRI done and the report said "multilevel spinal stenosis with disc prolapse L2/L3, consider surgical referral."

An enthusiastic and experienced silver-haired surgeon talked to Ric after the nurse practitioner took his history and did an examination. Ricardo learned that upper lumbar disc bulges are more common in middle-aged and older people than the young and they cause more backache than sciatica. It wasn't very big and wouldn't be hard to remove, but even a small disc hernia can sometimes cause big symptoms, partially due to the size of the nerve channels in the spine itself.

Ricardo also had spinal stenosis, which indicated that his nerve channels were quite narrow. They had likely been that way his whole life. It happens — some people are tall, some short, some have big nerve tunnels, some smaller. The surgeon said that this could be an issue in later life so why not relieve it at surgery too? It would mean a bit more time in the OR but overall should not change his post-op pain or recovery time much. *Sure, that makes sense.*

Surgery worked well and Ric got about five perfect years out of it before backache started up again. He found he could relieve it by stooping a bit. After a while, he saw his surgeon again, who advised he see an athletic therapist to make his back muscles stronger. That and his Tylenol did the job until he sold his flourishing business and retired at 67. By then he was stooping a lot.

For about a year after he retired, the backache eased a bit but never really went away. His stoop, on the other hand, was only increasing. Two years later Ric was bent enough to need a cane and was sore all the time. He had trouble being on his feet long enough to enjoy traveling so he stopped that. When his chiropractor couldn't help him, his family doctor advised physio, which just made him hurt more. So another MRI was done. More spinal stenosis, and referral to another surgeon.

HE'S BAAACK...

This surgeon took Ricardo's medical history and carefully examined the patient himself. Ric could pull himself up out of the stoop but not for very long, less than a minute. After finding that most of the muscles in Ric's legs were so weak that he could overpower them with his hands, the doctor asked him to try walking without his cane in the office a bit and he couldn't; every other step he was falling over. The surgeon ordered new X-rays and honestly Ric was looking forward to lying down on the X-ray stretcher, but this crazy doctor had him do the films standing up.

Back in the office Ricardo waited for quite some time while the doctor sat at his desk playing on his computer. Then he called his patient in. He frowned a lot.

First he brought up an MRI and showed it to Ricardo, explaining some basic anatomy and showing Ric bone, discs, things called *midline laminas* and *lateral bony facet joints* in the back of the spine, and the nerve sac in the middle of it all. Then he brought up another MRI and explained that this second scan was Ric's. This one looked very different. There was almost no nerve sac to be seen anywhere. In the other scan, it had been a long white streak running from top to bottom through the length of the scan images, and here all Ric saw was a lot of thick black bumps where the nerve sac should be. The surgeon explained that these were arthritically swollen facet joints that were pretty much filling the spinal canal.

How can this be? My old surgeon told me he had opened up my nerve channel with a bunch of "laminasomethings." Doesn't that mean he cut some bone away and opened my nerve tunnels?

The surgeon confirmed that the laminectomies were there on Ric's scan; they looked like little gaps in the posterior bone of the spine, and then he brought up a measuring cursor on the image software and measured them. They were small. Roughly 8 millimeters wide. The doctor explained that a normal nerve sac might be twice that size. There was exactly the opposite problem with the facet joints: they might normally be about 10 millimeters across and the cursor measured Ric's at almost 25. You could literally see the joints reaching the middle at some spots and seeming to rub on one another. The surgeon said from what he was looking at, it was a wonder that Ricardo could stand and walk at all.

He also explained that Ric had likely been protecting himself from catastrophe with the stoop. The volume of space available for the nerve sac varies greatly with posture, from a low point when we stand up straight and increasing as we bend forward. So Ric's stoop had been decompressing his nerves in much the same way that a surgeon might.

Next he pointed out the "mini X-ray" images on the scan — he called them *scanograms* — and explained that these were used to help focus the MRI scanner properly. They were little pictures of the length of Ric's spine, nice and straight from the front and smoothly curved when seen from the side.

Then he brought up the new standing X-rays that had just been done. They looked very different. From the front, Ricardo's spine — quite straight when he'd been comfy lying down in the MRI scanner — was now bent over to one side; the software measured a 35-degree scoliosis angle. From the side, Ric's low back was now almost perfectly straight and looking at the whole picture one could just about see how his body was pitched forward into the stoop. Here the doctor spent a few more minutes doing geometry with the angle measuring thing and literally popped out a *Wow!* He said that Ricardo was bent forward almost 65 degrees from a normal vertical position.

Doc explained that in simple terms Ric had multilevel recurrent translumbar lateral recess stenosis with high-grade cauda equina compression, post-laminectomy instability and sagittal plane imbalance with lumbopelvic mismatch. *Gesundheit!*

The surgeon declared Ric's spine "a disaster." "This is awful. I honestly don't know if I can fix it all. Trying, especially in a great big guy like you, might kill you if it doesn't kill me."

Ric had to ask, *How can this happen?*

WHAT HAD HAPPENED

The surgeon explained that because the spine is a linked kinetic chain, wear-and-tear degeneration is almost never focused at just one spot but scattered around everywhere. When a patient like this has an operation, the active problem operated on is fixed, but there is always a chance that something else in the spine can wear out and bring the patient back in the future. *Wish that other guy had told me that.*

Surgeon 2 didn't have the old pre-surgical scan or report to compare to but there was an OR note in the hospital computer that described the disc removal and the laminectomies. He wasn't happy with it and admitted he didn't understand why Ric had had laminectomies in the first place. He explained that the lamina is an important part of the stabilizing structure of the spine; a lot of the muscles and ligaments that hold us up and help our spine move around attach to it. With disc hernia, the lamina usually doesn't have to be completely removed; it only has to be thinned a bit to create space for the surgeon's tools to reach in and extract the disc. Most of it can be preserved. The previous surgeon had done not one but two *full* laminectomies to get the disc out, and then two more below it because there was reported to be "some stenosis" there.

That was a problem. The laminas cover the middle part of the spinal canal. But Ricardo's degenerative stenosis came from facet arthritis that was based laterally. The nerve channel became narrowed as the facets, gradually enlarging with arthritis (like a bunion), grew into the spinal canal from either side.

So why did I get better after the old surgery? For starters, Surgeon 1 did take the problem disc out. Secondly, there's a lining membrane deep to the lamina called the *ligamentum flavum* that connects to and covers the facet joints. Likely some of that was removed back then and that would have relieved a bit of pressure on the nerves but not much of it. That's what all the black stuff in the current scan is.

So why is my spine so bendy and stooped? Am I standing that way just to unpinch my nerves? In part yes but also no. If he really needed all that bend to decompress, Ric would be bent all the time, and there'd be no way he could lie flat in the scanner. Rick's spine was *unstable*, worn out like an arthritic knee that was so far gone the ligaments had stretched out and the knee would collapse when the person tried to stand on it.

Why is it unstable? Likely because of all those laminectomies. Laminectomy can weaken the spine a lot. Some research suggests a disc becomes twice as flexible as normal when the lamina behind it is removed. In the neck it's so common a problem that laminectomy is almost always supported by a screw/rod fusion done at the same time to prevent collapse. In the chest, the rib cage supports the spine and surgeons can usually get away with no fusion there, as long as they are careful not to trim out the adjacent facet joints too.

In the low back, laminectomy is very traditional and likely safe in the commonly operated lowermost levels where the spine arches backwards into the normal lumbar lordosis alignment — or hollow of the low back — which biomechanically protects one from collapsing forward. But laminectomy done at multiple levels, higher up the spine, would mean higher risk. No, Surgeon 2 wouldn't have done surgery as it had been done. If he'd been operating, he'd have removed all those enlarged facet joints and tossed some screws in there at the same time.

What's the lumbopelvic mismatch thing? Surgeon 2 explained that every spine has a certain ideal alignment that helps us comfortably stand up straight. Think about it: normally standing up straight is very easy and we can smoothly wobble around the usual standing posture a bit. But if we wobble enough, we'd fall over unless we tense up our back and our legs to pull ourselves back erect.

Anything beyond about 10 degrees off the ideal alignment increases people's pain and disability in a big way. Imagine trying to walk around all day bent forward by 10 degrees, you'd get backache in no time as your muscles started cramping to keep you from falling over. Ricardo's measurements showed that he was almost *65 degrees* out of alignment. Support from a cane or walker or wall-walking (leaning against the walls to hobble around the house) becomes necessary.

Can you straighten me up at surgery, Doc? Likely, at least in part. We should never expect spine surgery to make the patient "perfect," but we can generally make you much much better.

Spines most commonly collapse through disc degeneration and that was what Ricardo's had done. In simple terms, the spine has a "front" part where the discs are and a "back" part where the facet joints and laminas are. The neurological stuff is in the middle. Several of his discs were almost completely gone and so the vertebrae were rubbing bone on bone. That can be very painful and can throw alignment off completely. A normal disc in an average-sized person is about a half inch thick. Ric had collapsed all six, so even if he were perfectly aligned, he'd be three inches shorter now than God had made him.

There are a number of steps involved in figuring out how best to do the alignment correction. Lengthening the collapsed front part with a classical open incision quickly becomes Very Big Surgery and so it has become common practice to cut away some bone in the back (that's an osteotomy, of which there are a number of types), shortening the back to match the front. With an unstable spine, some of that disc collapse would likely correct "on the table" and then a fusion operation in that position (in situ) would give some correction. The trouble is, how do we *maintain* that correction?

We get the most robust support by operating right onto those disc spaces to put support devices called *cages* in there, and doing the bone graft fusion there too. Today a lot of that can be done with very nice minimally invasive technology. In these situations, I am a sort-of fan of anterior-approach MIS, which allows us to approach the discs through the belly or from the flank, but really I think it's all best done with an open incision and from the back because we have very good control of alignment changes that way and can be definitive in dealing with any stenosis.

There are surgical tools that help us elevate the collapsed disc spaces and recreate a more normal alignment while we're at it. Doing that in one disc space can correct alignment by maybe 5 to 10 degrees, and we might add a bit with a small shortening osteotomy at the same level. The bigger pedicle subtraction osteotomy might correct about 30 degrees.

But just one of those inside-the-disc-space interbody fusions can bleed as much as a person gives as a blood donor. Doing five or six can potentially add up to a person losing half their blood volume — if all goes well. In a great big man, we might double it. There was real potential for Ricardo to bleed out here.

Why is bleeding such a big thing in bigger patients? Spine surgery is different from most others because we have to dissect through the back muscle to get there. The back muscles are commonly several inches deep in a larger patient, and muscle is the most vascular (that is, bloody) major tissue we have. The biggest belly or chest or heart or brain surgery goes through very little muscle. This is why minimally invasive surgery (MIS) technology has real promise in spine care. Technology exists today to let us do all this without a major incision. But not every hospital has it.

During open spine surgery (using a major incision) we can do a lot to decrease that bleeding: the Jackson operating table was designed to lower the pressure in the veins of the spine. We can inject the muscle with epinephrine solutions that put blood vessels into spasm, and we can give intravenous or local blood-thickening drugs to help too (tranexamic acid is very popular), but still it can be an issue. If we ding the big blood vessels found immediately in front of the spine in these big deformity operations, it can be fatal.

Doing all this was huge surgery; it might be more than could safely be done in a day. Ric might need two or even three staged operations a few days apart. It might not even be doable at all if Ric bled too much or the scarring from previous surgery was overwhelming. Surgeon 2 said he'd just back off and close the wound if it came to that.

Still want to have back surgery? It's a bit more involved than just popping off to physio. Ricardo signed up.

For big surgery, we don't book two hours of OR time and the golf club an hour later. We book all day and really need to be at our best. No wine at dinner the night before, get to bed early and have a good breakfast.

This wasn't just big surgery; it was huge. The incision was almost a foot long. The flesh was almost six inches deep. It's hard just seeing down there to do the work in the first place!

Ric straightened out a lot on the OR table, everywhere but at the L4/L5 level which was his most "bent." Deformity correction would focus there — but this was more than a deformity case. There was all that "high-grade" spinal stenosis everywhere that needed decompressing. Extreme stenosis can be a big technical challenge even in a virgin spine, and here there was scar tissue from the old laminectomies that slowed down the work and increased the bleeding a great deal. All this work took five hours and bled enough to get anesthesia thinking about transfusion as they gave the second dose of IV antibiotics, routinely due at four hours. The team scrubbed out for a break, a pee and a snack (yeah, sometimes we do that) and to look over some in-the-OR X-rays to decide on what was next and how much more to do.

That L4/L5 was still awfully collapsed, but overall the spine was much straighter already, about 20 degrees worth. Doing an inter-body fusion with posterior release osteotomy at L4/L5 would likely correct at least another 10 or 15 degrees, and each level of simple posterior "shortening" osteotomy above that might give another five or 10 apiece. It's not ideal. We know deformity is best corrected at the lower two levels of the spine, but even with the best of knowledge and technology available one still needs to be reasonable. That wasn't bad and likely enough surgery in one day for both the team and the patient.

Research data suggests that if the spine patient is in the OR for more than about eight hours, the risk of many complications skyrockets. Some hospitals deliver megasurgery with several teams of surgeons working one after the other, but most don't have that capability. Not every hospital can do this work and not every surgeon can do it either. If need be, the team could come back another day, accomplishing the reconstruction in two staged procedures.

The interbody fusion at L4/L5 went well and improved alignment there a lot. Then the surgeons drove 14 screws into the spine and another two big "bolts" into the pelvis below it before hooking up the rods. Not two rods but four rods — in surgery like this, the terrific force on a standard rod can break it as much as 15 percent of the time, so a smart surgeon supplements it.

Surgery's done. Wash out the wound a few times, make sure nothing's bleeding. Sewing up all that flesh can take another hour. Almost 10 hours skin to skin. Park the patient in ICU overnight just to be on the safe side. Anybody who's received five units of blood has great potential to get sick in a number of ways.

HOW IT TURNED OUT

Ricardo did great. You'd think surgery like this would just about kill the patient but the opposite is commonly true. These people are so badly off beforehand that even with the raw wound still bleeding, they are often smiling and happy as soon as they wake up. No kidding.

Ric was up in a chair the day after surgery, stood with his walker the day after that and physio had to adjust his walker because straightening out his spine had made him almost four inches taller already! So happy! Stronger legs, sciatic pains all gone, easier to stand with his straighter spine.

All that surgically dissected muscle bleeds and oozes internally for several days after surgery, so the surgeon inserted a wound drain while closing and it sucked out bloody stuff for several days. Ricardo needed transfusions of several units of blood over those days to maintain a reasonable blood count. His fluid and electrolyte metabolism also went bonkers, so the team worked to normalize all that too.

The surgeon put him in a brace. There's no academic research anywhere to say that shows a benefit to the spine's alignment, but common sense should tell us that anything we can do to encourage that patient to hold themselves as erect as possible might minimize the risk of a post-op collapse of the operated spine, especially in deformity cases where the patient has been "preprogrammed" to bend forward and there's often osteoporosis. Yes, that happens; screws can tear loose and rods break and cage implants can actually be crushed down into the vertebrae they're supporting, especially when the high loads of bending forward and twisting are applied before the bone graft fusions have had time to heal strongly (which seems to take a minimum of three or four months — just like your badly broken arm or leg does). The surgeon told Ric he wanted him wearing his brace for six months, whenever he was up.

The broken-ankle patient almost always protects themselves after surgery. One look at their purple swollen foot and the brain knows not to jump around on it before it looks really, really normal. Because the spine is "back there," out of sight and therefore out of mind, it often gets abused once the pain of the cut is gone. If nothing else, wearing the brace is a daily reminder to the patient to behave themselves and protect their back from postural overloads. The only thing worse than doing surgery like this is having to do it a second time.

A year and a half later Ric was very happy: pain free, standing straight and able to enjoy travel. He was even back in the pool he loved to swim in! X-rays showed his corrected alignment had held up pretty well; the surgery had given him almost 40 degrees of angular correction and his imbalance was just under 25 degrees, abnormal by the textbook but more than acceptable to him. Those X-rays still looked far from perfect and they made the surgeon squirm, but the patient was happy with symptom relief and that's the name of the game, isn't it?

SPINE CRIMES

Doing several contiguous laminectomies and not discussing the chance of a structural collapse with the patient is a spine crime that should never happen.

Seeing such a patient having difficulty standing up and telling him to strengthen his back without examining him at all or taking even a basic X-ray? Another spine crime.

Proposing or planning surgery in this day and age without getting pre-op X-rays and, especially in a lumbar case, not getting those X-rays done in the standing position? A third spine crime. Outside of major research centers and lead academic spine care facilities, standing X-rays seem to be rare even today but research shows a third of spinal stenosis patients go out of alignment as soon as the patient stands up! Sadly, relying on only traditional X-rays and MRIs — both done with the patient lying down — is still very common. For Ricardo, that would have been disastrous as the MRI might have indicated another simple decompression operation, removing structure in the bony facet joints and almost certainly rendering his already unstable spine even more unstable.

Chapter 22

My Top 20 Tips for the Successful Spine Surgeon (and Their Patients)

This list of spine care essentials is more pointedly surgical and, therefore, more technical than the corresponding list for primary care practitioners and their patients at the end of Part I. The more specialized subject matter that follows is aimed at helping my surgeon colleagues who are not spine specialists avoid the missed diagnoses and poor treatment outcomes that come from our own ranks all too often.

This is material that, again, every potential spine surgery patient should know about as they might work towards decisions about their surgical care. When my patient grills me on details of surgery, sure, I instinctively tend to get my back up a bit as all physicians commonly do. But I work hard to control that, and after I listen well and explain things to the patient, we generally end up with a more satisfactory outcome (for both of us!) when all is said and done. My hope is that with both surgeon and patient armed with this information, the results will be better for all concerned.

1. **Take a history. Yourself.** This step should not just be delegated to trainees, PAs or nurse clinicians without

direct supervision or detailed review. It takes five minutes, just four more than asking, "What hurts?" If you do want to delegate, your potential delegates should work alongside you for at least two or three months to learn how it's done properly. Teach them the essentials of assessment and diagnosis, including that the manual motor examination is as insensitive as we know it to be; that the key symptom in lumbar stenosis is not pain or numbness or weakness but claudication; and that we have to ask probing questions when many patients just say they hurt.

2. **Don't be planning the OR when you first meet the patient.** Most acute spines get better without surgery, and most chronic ones don't evolve quickly. So conservative care and deferral go first in most cases.

3. **Don't be algorithmic.** Because outcomes from surgery to relieve sciatica are felt to be so much more consistent than surgery to alleviate back pains, too many surgeons teach and practice that back pain itself can never be treated at all and therefore deny their back pain patients care. Don't be that doctor. Consistently, the spine-fusions literature even in "nonspecific" back pain shows that about two-thirds of patients get good benefit from this surgery, relieving their pain symptoms and improving their quality of life. That's at least as good as our best research outcomes on lumbar stenosis from the landmark research Spine Patient Outcomes Research Trial (SPORT) in spinal stenosis.

Sure, the "chronic pain" patient who's been sore for just seven weeks should be cautious about having major surgery, but when you meet patients who have been in pain and disabled for years and who have failed extensive nonoperative care, giving them a two out of three chance of relief from their lives of misery may not be a bad option.

4. **Get your pain patients to take a finger and point exactly to where it hurts, first thing.** This helps you focus on where the problem is and what it might be. You will learn a lot more about the problem — and you will be more likely to make an accurate diagnosis — if you have the patient *show* you precisely where it hurts rather than having them just *tell* you about the pain.

5. **Have your patient stand up and walk a bit.** We can get a lot of hints as to what's wrong from posture and gait even when the bedside motor exam is normal. In fact, the manual motor physical examination for weakness is very insensitive. Basic biomechanics reminds us we put 3.5 body weights' joint reactive force across hip, knee and ankle in simple walking, and our leg muscles have to be terrifically powerful to control all that. A few pounds of manual resistance at the bedside exam isn't powerful enough to detect any deficit. Many patients with profound neurological dysfunction aren't in fact weak enough to be diagnosed in the manual motor exam, but on their feet there could be clear evidence of their deficits.

6. **Know what different deficits are telling you.** Drop foot is usually no great crisis. It's primarily an L5 deficit. When chronic it's often a minor disability easily accommodated with a limp or a splint. It gets more press than most motor nerve root deficits likely because the ankle dorsiflexors are the smallest and weakest major motor unit in our leg and, therefore, often the first deficit to be detected manually. L3 (and sometimes L4) deficits make people's knees buckle and S1 does the same at the ankle so these have much more important

implications, causing ambulatory impairment generally and an increased risk of falls in the elderly. The old "get-up-and-go" test is a great quads screen. For S1 deficit your patient has to be able to do a toe raise — in single stance, because tandem toe raise misses a lot!

7. **Get your X-rays done standing up to improve diagnostic accuracy.** Spine alignment can change substantially from the lying down position, and standing X-rays detect more instability than old-style flexion/extension views do. One in three lumbar spinal stenosis patients has some spondylolisthesis that's only evident in standing films and will appear to be aligned normally in the common supine X-rays or MRI.

8. **In the lumbar spine, use simple laminectomy only for true bony central spinal stenosis, which is rare.** Degenerative stenosis is usually based laterally and easily treated with lateral recess decompressions that preserve the midline tension band and biomechanical stability.

9. **If there's any baseline malalignment or instability at all, if you have to do aggressive bilateral facet resection, or the motion segment is very hypermobile in the OR after your decompression, just whack some screws in there to keep your patient out of trouble.** We should almost never do "fusion for spinal stenosis" as a standalone; that shouldn't be a thing because it doesn't make sense. Do a fusion for (1) baseline instability or unacceptable deformity, (2) anticipated instability after major posterior column resection, and (3) vertically collapsed foramena where the motion segment has to be elevated with interbody fusion implants to decompress the nerve root there.

10. **Beware the "tall" disc where post-laminectomy instability may be most likely.** Mobility — and so the potential for instability — will likely be greatest with a healthy mobile

disc. When your patient's discs are all eroded and there's bone-on-bone pseudo-articulation in the anterior column +/- osteophytes, things will be much more stable.

11. **Always be cautious about uninstrumented laminectomy.** It is generally OK in the mid and upper thoracic spine where the chest wall contributes 40 percent of the spine's stability, but avoid it or consider instrumenting it even if it's at the apex of physiological kyphosis. Be cautious distally in the T-spine where the spine rotates in the lower thoracic segments, and opposite the relatively mobile upper three lumbar vertebrae. Remember laminectomy is different from facet resection. Particularly with metastatic tumor, if there's a lot of facet resection needed, we should have a low threshold to instrument.

12. **Almost nobody does a simple laminectomy in the neck because of the known risk for post-laminectomy kyphosis, but we take that risk in the lumbar spine all the time — I'd ask why?** Laminectomy increases the flexion strain or "bendability" of a lumbar motion segment by 130 percent. Classical laminectomies were in the majority done at lower levels where the spine is lordotic, relatively immobile and so protected from flexion instability. If your patient is kyphotic at baseline, be aware of this risk. And again, beware the "tall" disc — collapsed discs seem to be much less prone to post-decompressive instability or recurrent disc prolapse.

13. **Think about spine sagittal balance all the time, with every low back and neck case in particular.** Don't be the academic colleague (and teacher!) who was recently heard to say, "I don't care about kyphosis," and whose practice outcomes reflect that. Sure, we have decades of literature saying that a simple in-situ fusion can be a great thing, but most of that literature predates what we know about spinal alignment today. Data suggest that

improving or even correcting malalignment at fusion will likely give your patient a better long-term outcome. And data shows that by doing so you may cut the odds of your patient needing more work in the future!

14. **Understand the three-part anatomy of the lateral recess,** deal with all of it to thoroughly decompress your stenosis patient and don't expect facetectomy to decompress a vertically collapsed infrapedicular recess (or even the foramen, unless you've gone proximally enough to visualize and dissect the undersurface of the exiting root). This pathoanatomy needs either elevation of the collapsed motion segment (with an interbody implant or distractive pedicle screw instrumentation), or resection of the offending collapsed pedicle. Some might say an interspinous process device might work, but I am not a fan, especially if collapse is asymmetric (degenerative scoliosis).

15. **Understand some elementary biomechanics and use that knowledge to ask your patients to avoid flexion posture for a while after surgery, or even permanently.** Flexion dramatically increases the compression load on our discs, and likely the coaxial pullout stress on our implants. I like three months; most recurrent lumbar disc prolapse seems to happen that early and it takes that long for your fusion to start consolidating too. There's no hard proof of benefit to this common sense concept, but in all my years I have done very few acute recurrent discs or revisions for loose screws from my own practice.

16. **Beware the lumbar stenotic with preserved ankle and knee-jerk reflexes.** The lumbar stenosis patient should present like a flaccid lower motor neuron disease. Preserved reflexes may be a clue to tandem cervical stenosis and masked myelopathy.

17. **Think about antibiotics after surgery.** Allegedly one pre-op dose is enough but our traditional "best evidence" on this is very poor-quality evidence. If you don't believe me, read the North American Spine Society guideline document (available on their website, spine.org). Wound biology says the first "inflammatory phase" of wound healing takes about three days, so it likely takes that time for a fresh wound to become bacteriostatic. You put antibiotic ointment and a Band-Aid on your own cut finger for a couple of days, why not treat your patients with the same basic common sense? I routinely prescribe for 48 hours, even giving my ambulatory cases a few days of oral antibiotics in their exit prescription. I give IV antibiotics to my inpatient cases for 72 hours if there's immune compromise from steroids, diabetes, frailty or obesity. My practice data here are still evolving but it looks good!

18. **Antibiotic resistance is a good thing to avoid.** We see lots of people who vaguely report themselves as allergic to penicillin and so we treat with alternative antibiotics. I don't believe an extra day or two of penicillin (as discussed above) is a bad thing but the widespread use of second- and third-generation drugs likely is. Why not take the time to screen the allergy symptom history or send them to an allergist pre-op to minimize our use of alternative drugs that might eventually lead to more aggressive resistance? Or just delve into the "allergic" history? Data confirm that unless there's a clearly defined history of major reaction (hives or anaphylaxis), the risk of major allergy is trivial.

19. **If your neurological compression patient has just pain, without major motor strength loss or functional impairment, there are a lot of nonsurgical pain care options to try.** As long as the patient is taught to know

what the symptoms of neurological deterioration are and is reliable enough to report them, that's fine. However, if the patient has a *disabling* motor/functional deficit at presentation, it's hard to argue with the known benefit of surgical decompression, and that care should be delivered sooner rather than later.

20. **If your neurological patient isn't significantly better or at least different after surgery, consider reimaging right away to make sure they're thoroughly decompressed.** If by three months, and certainly by six, they're not very seriously improved, work them up again to make sure both that they've been thoroughly decompressed and that there aren't other comorbidities like peripheral vascular disease, neuropathy or appendicular arthritis confounding recovery.

Part 3

Spine Care Solutions

*In which we are presented possible — and
realistic — ways to improve spine care.*

Chapter 23
First and Foremost — Education!

Most doctors don't get much learning in spine care.

What, in the majority, do we do today when something comes up and we don't know much about it? We Google it! Before Google, we *learned* about it.

Googling and learning are very different things. Googling can help one to *know* something in the instant — and that can be very helpful for a physician. I do it all the time, for example when I come across some drug that my patient is taking that I've never heard of before. But to *learn* about that drug, I'd have to study its pharmacology and chemistry, side effects and interactions, and that takes some time.

With lots and lots of learning, eventually we might come to *understand* something. That's the pinnacle of medical practice capability, a form of what we call wisdom. It's a very real thing. In every hospital, in every discipline, everybody knows who the "go-to" person is. For a long time at my hospital, in the fields of internal medicine and intensive care, Dr. "Keep 'Em Alive" Clive Davis was felt by many of us to have a direct line to God. Of course he didn't; he'd just been doing what he did for a long time with unusual intensity and dedication and simply knew more about these practice areas than anybody else in the place.

Physicians today are driven to be "lifelong learners"; the practice and knowledge base of health care are evolving all the time, and if we don't work to stay current, we get dated very fast. Historically, it was possible for a physician to go into practice after basic specialty training and never learn a thing again. True story: long ago, when I was interviewing for jobs, a potential colleague told me, "I haven't opened a book for eight years." His practice showed it, and his patients suffered for it. Today things are very different. Most of us are required to do a certain amount of Continuing Medical Education (CME) every year to maintain our licenses and we do, but sadly a lot of that "education" really amounts to an overpriced holiday somewhere sunny where we may or may not attend a single lecture.

In all of this, most physicians get virtually no spine care education at all. At my own institution, most graduating medical students have been exposed in their core training to just one backache case review and 11 PowerPoint slides with the word *spine* on them before going on to specialty training and practice. That's a problem. One simply cannot have any basic knowledge at all if one has never been exposed to a thing in a meaningful way. I, for example, took a computer science course way back in the '80s, complete with punch cards and an IBM mainframe, but I know zero about modern digital computer coding and am very weak in tech generally. (Trying to figure out Dropbox and Wix took my stress levels off the charts! Surgery is soooo much easier.)

Spine care might be considered a part of musculoskeletal (MSK) care generally, and even MSK is simply not a significant thing in the modern undergraduate medical curriculum. Shockingly, only 15 percent of U.S. med schools even *have* an MSK curriculum despite the fact that 20 percent of patient visits to the doctor relate to MSK complaints! Within MSK, spine is the biggest and fastest growing care field — and we don't learn (or teach) it to any great extent! The modern medical student knows this. When asked in surveys how comfortable they are with handling MSK issues, most report that they are not.

Spine care today is a monster, a huge field of practice, and it's a very costly monster. The February 2022 issue of the *Journal of Bone and Joint Surgery* (jbjs.org) features a research article and a commentary on this topic, from which we learn that spine has become the single biggest cost item in U.S. health care, apparently $135 billion worth in 2016 and still growing! So shouldn't we teach our doctors a bit about it? MSK practitioners know and recognize that inadequate spine care and education about the spine are big issues, but we have no real way to drive them forward. The medical curriculum is very full with cancer and cardiovascular care and all the more classical things doctors are felt to need knowledge of, so to add to it without lengthening the training, we'd have to cut something else out — what would it be?

IMPROVING THE GENERAL PHYSICIAN'S KNOWLEDGE OF — AND COMFORT WITH — ELEMENTARY SPINE CARE

The lack of knowledge in the body of physicians who refer patients to me and with whom I practice has been a concern for me for a long time and so I've done a few small things to address the problem locally where I practice, things like lecturing at grand rounds in several disciplines and giving talks at specialty education days. It's not a huge thing to deliver some elementary but thorough learning on the major issues in just a short lecture. Every time I do it, I get a lot of "Wow! Thanks, I never knew that!" But I can't possibly get to everybody. At McMaster, I've actually had discussions with administrators about doing a spine lecture in medical training programs where I'd say learners need it most, say family medicine, internal medicine, neurology and physiatry.

I think that if there was *just one day* devoted to spine learning in the general medical curriculum, we could change for the better the outcomes and prognoses for many patients.

It would be entirely possible in just one day to educate medical students to the point where many of the disasters I've presented in this book could be avoided through earlier recognition and referral to care. I know it's possible to cover that much important ground in such a short time. The lecture's pretty much built and I've delivered it successfully at many of the multidisciplinary talks I've given, in a lot less time than a full day.

And the education gap lies not only within our universities and colleges. The spine academic and professional societies fail themselves, and our patients, here as well. All of them offer a regular menu of learning activities to us members . . . but we already know most of this stuff! They are preaching to the choir of highly trained spine specialists and surgeons, but none of them seem to offer a curriculum directed to the general medical or paramedical spine care practitioner. Every one of the elite spine care societies ought to promote spine care training opportunities beyond their membership.

Outside of that, I'd like to see every specialist spine surgeon like myself give a lecture on elementary spine care to their local physician base even just once a year.

Obviously, I'm a dreamer. I'd like to change my world. I know that I can't do it on my own. But maybe, just maybe, some med school dean or a national curriculum planner somewhere will read this book and see the need I'm presenting. If that happens, the spine care world would become a better place and so many patients would have better outcomes.

IMPROVING SURGICAL CARE

This part gets tricky, and very political very fast. Medicine is a business, a very big business, and big business is always political. No matter how well-motivated the person in the white coat in front of you is, there are bureaucrats and institutions lined up behind them influencing and leveraging practice, and those are hard to change.

My teachers used to say that it took a surgeon five years of practice just to figure out what they really like to do, and another five years to get good at it. We've since knocked off some of that first five years with fellowship requirements for specialty training. A surgeon today very much has to decide what they want to do while still learning elementary stuff, many years before applying for highly competitive fellowships . . . but that second five years is a problem.

Malcolm Gladwell in his remarkable book *Outliers* discusses definitions of expertise, and it seems one needs about 10,000 hours of dedicated learning to get really good at something. A 50-week year of 40-hour workweeks is just 2,000 hours, so expertise needs five years. Standard orthopedics residency training is five years long, so we're good there. But. When I'm training a fellow in spine surgery, I feel strongly that it takes me two full years of additional clinical training to bring that person to the point where they *start* to understand the spine and are ready to go forward with a life of learning towards true expertise.

Unfortunately, spine fellowship specialty training still doesn't have any widely recognized curriculum. There's no board certification in spine like there is in orthopedics or neurosurgery. Most fellows today do two years in all. One is a largely nonclinical research year where they have to pump out scientific publications and get research grants that support the host university, and the other is clinical — so they might get 2,000 hours of real surgery training, not enough by a long shot.

We could change that with a well-defined training curriculum and certification (that is, board exams in spine), but there's a great resistance to that in the medical marketplace. Today, every generally qualified orthopedic and neurosurgery graduate is licensed to practice spine surgery, and nobody wants to give that up. We've tried. There was an American Board of Spine Surgery running a qualifying exam for some time (that organization has folded into the North American Spine Society, I believe), but when they went to the U.S. medical authorities for recognition as a specialty, they were shut down by lobbying from the established disciplines. Europe is ahead here: there's a group of academic surgeons and others who've defined the European Economic Community e-learning curriculum in spine (eccelearning.com). I think it's a wonderful thing. Several European countries have apparently ratified it and require surgeons to complete that complex (and expensive!) learning curriculum before they can practice at the speciality spine care hospital.

There's an analogy to be made here to surgery of the hand. As in spine surgery where orthopedics and neurosurgery intersect, elements of hand surgery are done by orthopedists (bone work), neurosurgeons (nerves, obviously) and plastic surgeons (tendons and ligaments). For decades, an American surgeon who has a dedicated practice in any one of these disciplines has been able to write a board exam and be certified as a specialist hand surgeon. Why not do the same in spine?

Even without going that far, we *could* easily require a new spine surgeon to be audited, to include an element of supervised practice to ensure that standards in spine care are being met. Theoretically, when a surgeon joins a hospital now, the first year or so is often "on probation," meaning somebody makes sure they know what they're doing and are safe and good at it before they permanently join the hospital staff. But too often that doesn't happen — remember the *Dr. Death* series that streamed on Peacock and Showcase? Practically speaking, the new guy gets all the bad on-call days and underpaid or uninsured cases, commonly working unsupervised and unaudited while everybody else relaxes and has a good time doing the easy stuff. Often the new guys quite frankly dodge us, likely because they don't want to seem lacking in expertise or confidence.

I can't remember when a newbie last asked me for an opinion or help with a case . . . and too often they should have.

I'd like to see a system where a newbie surgeon is paired with somebody very senior for that first year, working one-on-one for every case and every consult. Just by billing the assist fees, the newbie will earn a good living and it would be a great way for some of that "wisdom" thing to be passed along too. Then for the second year, the senior is tasked with reviewing all the junior surgeon's surgery and outcomes to make sure things continue to go well.

So far all I've talked about goes to the start of surgical practice. Remember lifelong learning? I'd like to see more aggressive enforcement there too. Way too often surgeons amass their credits in the Caribbean (or some other nice place) at marginal meetings where learning is scanty. In spine we have several recognized lead academic societies where the annual meetings are a wonderful learning experience. In North America, it's the North American Spine Society (duh! spine.org); in Europe, it's AO Spine (aospine .org) or EUROSPINE (eurospine.org); the UK has BritSpine (ukssb.com); and there are others around the world. I'd like to see it be a part of credentialing that a spine surgeon attend at least one of these leading academic meetings in the spine care field every year, *in addition* to their country's other baseline CME requirements.

My spine teachers used to say spine care can be as seamless and predictable as slamming in a hip or knee replacement (I know surgeons who do five or six of those in a day), or zipping out your gallbladder or appendix (ditto). Nobody's terrified about having those procedures done, but almost every spine surgery patient is scared to death! My field has a terrible reputation because of primary care and surgical issues like those I've shared with you in this book. My teachers taught that the spine care patient needs the right diagnosis and the right procedure delivered at the right time. When that happens, surgical spine care really can be like every other operation.

Somewhere out there is my fantasy world where your spine care problem is diagnosed early for what it is and referred promptly to a caring, qualified surgeon who has adequate training and resources to deliver excellent care in a safe, efficient, effective and timely way. I'm still dreaming. Share my hope!

Chapter 24
Common Red Flags in Spine Care

Know the signs of bad spine trouble.

There have always been clinical circumstances that can alert a doctor (or an informed patient) to potentially critical spine care problems, like a fracture or tumor or neurological compression. We vaguely teach them but there's no hard-and-fast truth here, for two reasons I think. One is that whenever science is applied to the concept, it doesn't stand up to analysis because "false positives" — signs of trouble when it's not there — are very common. False negatives or "misses" happen too. Another reason that no red flags list is written in stone is that no professional association is bold enough to support such a list due to the potential liability implications. In my opinion, none of that means we shouldn't discuss them. I'd rather see 10 cases referred for signs of trouble that didn't pan out than miss just one really critical one. So, here goes . . .

1. **Pain that comes on spontaneously, with no history of injury.** Aches and sprains don't do that. Tumors, infections and osteoporosis fractures do though.

2. **Pain that is not relieved by rest (lying down).** Certainly some instabilities and deformity pain are relieved this way, but the neurological compressions are not.

3. **Pain that is rapidly growing in intensity despite increasing doses of powerful analgesics.** Duh. Most cases of spinal stenosis and degenerative neurological compressions don't evolve quickly, but tumors and infections and cauda equina syndrome can and do.

4. **Pain focused in the mid-back or thoracic region, from the base of the neck and opposite the ribs.** We sprain and strain our necks and low back all the time. Not so much the mid-back. Pain here could be caused by something more serious, especially when it lasts more than a week or two.

5. **Pain in the back or legs associated with a burning sensation.** Backache doesn't burn; neurological or neuropathic pain commonly does.

6. **Severe pain that comes on very suddenly, often after injury, like a fall or bending or stretching too far.** Until proven otherwise, that's likely a disc hernia or a fracture.

7. **Lasting pain associated with weight loss.** Could be a cancer, either in the spine or close to it.

8. **Lasting pain associated with hot flashes and cold chills.** Could be infection.

9. **In the legs, symptoms of pain, weakness or numbness that are worsened with standing erect or walking and relieved by bending forward.** (We call this *flexion rest* or the *shopping cart sign* — Google it!) This is claudication and could be a symptom of spinal stenosis.

10. **In the hands and arms, numbness that is constantly present** — not just at night or brought on in specific positions. It is a common early symptom of spinal cord compression in the neck. Sometimes there's a loss of

fine motor control in the hands as well; people feel like they're wearing gloves, so handwriting and texting become difficult and they drop things.

If you are a primary care provider, and your patient complains about any of these symptoms, they may warrant further investigation. These cases may not be just patients complaining of backache; there is a good chance that something serious — and potentially treatable — underlies pain that presents in any of these ways.

And if you are a patient experiencing any of these symptoms, be a strong advocate for yourself — insist that your doctor and other medical providers take your pain seriously. Give them as much information as you can; ask for diagnostic tests and push for referrals to specialists if need be. If nothing else, this book should have made it clear by now that sometimes your back pain is not just another annoying backache.

Chapter 25

Low Back and Neck Basics for the Patient

With tips and tricks for either staying well or managing your spine well enough to avoid care entirely.

One way to deal with the difficult problem of widespread practitioner ignorance in spine care would be to keep everybody's spine healthy in the first place. Hmm, not so easy. We know *some* people have a genetic predisposition to early spine degeneration, so even if we could perfectly eliminate the five simple risk factors for trouble beyond that, I'd have some work.

So like every other spine book out there, here's my pitch. For $99.95 go to www.magic_cure.com (geez, I hope that's not a thing) and buy my foolproof exercise program . . . People, that's not me, never has been and never will be. There's a bazillion exercise programs and other "prevention" treatments out there that don't work well no matter how much you pay for them. I'm too stupid to try to sell you one and so will likely be working for a living until I die.

Reader, this will be a bigger chapter because I have to explain a lot to justify what I'll tell you. The advice I'll offer you here is exactly what I give my patients. What I do may be considered unorthodox by many, and it is in the general world of spine care, but it's based on very sound biomechanics and anatomy and it works well. My patients generally do well with it and it's helped me avoid spine surgeons for 30 years myself.

WHAT YOU SHOULD UNDERSTAND TO HELP PROTECT YOURSELF FROM INJURY

Your spine is largely a skeletal structure, but it's different from the rest of the skeleton in that it's all about stability, not mobility. Arms and legs need lots of rehab after injuries or surgery to get functional range of motion back, but in the majority of cases, spines don't need that. Your spine has to hold balance to keep you erect all through the long day of supporting the huge biomechanical loads there. But the skeletal spine itself has no stability at all — stack up the bones in the anatomy lab and they fall right over! A spine needs the fleshy "back" around it to have great strength and endurance.

Especially endurance. Just standing up we don't realize our back muscles have to put out roughly a full body weight's force to hold us up, and we might be standing for hours on end. Arms and legs generally do only short-term "burst" activity — step, reach or grab. Try tightening up your thigh muscles real hard and holding it for an hour or so . . . nobody can do that! What your back muscles have to do is *different*. Stretching and yoga and massage to "break up the knots" in your back muscles will never give you that endurance strength.

The spine is designed to be internally mobile — a series of independent vertebrae connected by discs and facet joints, surrounding the spinal cord and a series of nerves — but it turns out that the *stability* of that entire structure is far more important. Consider idiopathic scoliosis, a twisting deformity most common in young teenagers that often sees them needing screw-and-rod fusions done along most of the length of their spine. After surgery, their spine *can't* move. Those kids go on to live their lives without, in most cases, any great disability or accelerated degeneration of their spines. There's a similar thing in older adults where the low back wears out so badly it collapses into a degenerative scoliosis. Those people commonly need fusions that go roughly "bra line to bum" (most of these cases are women). A lot of my little old ladies, once they've had about six months post-op to fuse and recover, can actually touch their toes! Which I can't do; I've always been a bit stiff.

How can this be, you ask? How can surgically rendering a spine (or part of it) immobile be beneficial when it is naturally mobile? Well, the same thing happens naturally in the human body. Muscles, and muscle spasm, stiffen the whole body in an attempt to provide stability and protect whatever hurts from moving around and hurting more, sacrificing mobility in the process. The back muscles originate as small things way up on the middle ribs between and just below your shoulder blades, then get bigger and broader as they span the hollow of your low back to connect to the pelvis below your waistline and just above your bum — effectively below the rotation point of your hips. When your back hurts, the muscles spasm to keep painful stuff in your spine from wobbling, and that spasm locks up your hips so your body won't bend forward, keeping you as erect and immobile as possible.

Yes, Virginia, back muscle spasm is often a *good* thing because it's protecting you from what wants to hurt more. It's not a primary problem but secondary one, a sign of an underlying issue, and it should prompt your caregivers to find your correct diagnosis.

Back muscle spasm explains why young trauma patients who have suffered a spine fracture, and most commonly break just below their rib cage at the top of the hollow of the low back, all complain of pain at the *bottom* when they're getting active again after care. The large, strong low back muscles weaken rapidly after the injury due to a few months of lessened activity while the fractures heal, and then the patients get muscle aches as they're gaining their strength back.

It also explains why some low back patients complain that their pain goes all the way up to their shoulder blades. I was taught those patients were nuts and blew off many people early in my career after scanning them up there and never finding any skeletal trouble. I was ignorant then, and I was wrong. Some patients for unclear reasons get spasm pain at the upper end of the back muscles where they originate as small muscle bands coming off the mid-thoracic vertebra and ribs. Although the real issue with their spine is in their lower back. I now know this firsthand as I get some pain there occasionally after a long surgery when my own low back injury is acting up.

TOP FIVE RISK FACTORS FOR LOW BACK TROUBLE, AND MAYBE SPINE ISSUES GENERALLY

Joe Cave Man was designed to live around 30 years, which is when even today we start to lose muscle mass and hormone levels drop off. He'd slow down a bit trying to run away and the lions would get him, end of story. Today we commonly live three times that long, so our spines are exposed to many more "load cycles" of bending and twisting and whatnot than evolution or God designed them for. It makes sense to do what we can to ease the pressure of all those loads and the accumulating microtrauma injury that comes with that (more to come, stay tuned).

The five risk factors that are known to accelerate disc degeneration (at least, in the low back) are quite simple and they all go to issues of long-term mechanical overloading of the spine:

1. Being very overweight
2. Heavy physical work with a lot of bending, leaning forward and/or twisting
3. Regular exposure to low-frequency motor vibrations (like a diesel engine or a Harley)
4. Smoking (which weakens the body's ability to heal any injury)
5. High levels of stress (the cortisol-type stress hormones do the same thing)

Reader, you should know that there's a world of literature on spine injury prevention and health out there, bags of research. Never anything definitive. There are lots of studies claiming "statistical significance," which in Science Talk means "this should be considered as proof"... but if that were true of the preventive advice they all offer, why hasn't anything presented in the scientific literature in my 40 years of spine care come out as truly effective? Because none of it really works.

In health care, most of the time we don't have rock-solid proof that a treatment is effective and so a smart practitioner has to go to the biology of the problem. Thorough understanding of that biology allows us to help the patient with basic preventive measures and treatments that can really make a difference.

Earlier I told you I learned long ago that most acute spine care conditions have a benign natural history, meaning they get better all by themselves. That's still true. But awhile into my training we learned that some of those back pain cases would have a second acute episode, then a third and a fourth. *Why is that?* we might ask.

I don't think it's because so many people have a naturally rotten, weak back. I think it's because people are never taught how to protect themselves against injury and so they keep reinjuring themselves. I believe that if you understand the spine's mechanical issues, you can very effectively protect yourself and stay away from pain for a very long time. I've done it for almost 30 years now myself.

In Las Vegas there's a hotel called New York-New York that has a roller coaster on the roof. It takes a big dip over the side of the building. In my 30s I was terrified on the thing and not braced well in my seat, my back unsupported as I cowered and slid my bum forward a bit, my body bowstringing across the seat. When we hit the first big dip at the bottom, something went *crunch*! I haven't been the same since.

My own problem, I think, is ILDD, internal lumbar disc derangement. (I have no proof; without unacceptable disability or a need to seek treatment, I haven't had the scans.) My problem is very mechanical. When I bend forward and turn left, I know about it immediately.

So I don't. I'm careful about almost every move I make, I pay religious attention to posture . . . and have had only four short flareups in 30 years. You can do that well too! How? By watching your posture. *Posture posture posture!* Here's some more history.

THE IMPORTANCE OF GOOD POSTURE

Back in the 1960s, a pioneer spine researcher called Alfred Nachemson did some amazing work with his patients that would likely never get past an ethics committee today. He surgically inserted pressure sensors into the discs of his awake, walking and talking patients via great big steel pins drilled through the skin into the back and had them stand, sit, bend and lie down with the pins sticking out to see what the pressures did. His research has stood the test of time and tells us a great deal about spine biomechanics and loads in different postures. (You can find it listed in the References section at the end of the book.)

Most commonly, spines deteriorate through disc degeneration. So to stay healthy we want to take loads off the discs *before* they get hurt . . . and certainly once they've been damaged a bit, like mine.

Remember the discs are small, at best about an inch and a half in diameter and half an inch thick. When healthy and young they're terrifically strong under load, stronger in fact than the bone around them. If a strongman could do a 10,000-pound deadlift, he wouldn't get a disc hernia; instead, the hydraulically tensed discs would fracture the bones between them. Young healthy people do that in blunt trauma accidents like car wrecks and falls all the time.

Remember the spine has a "front" part where the discs that carry the most load and vertebral bodies are, a "middle" where the neurological stuff is and a "back" or posterior part where the bony facet joints keep us aligned. So it makes sense, and Nachemson proved, that when we bend or lean forward, the loads on our discs increase dramatically, and when we recline or lie down, they drop. Nachemson found that when we're standing straight, the midlumbar discs carry almost 80 percent of our body weight in load (the facets would carry the rest). Leaning forward, later research suggests the loads almost quadruple! When we sit, even in a straight-backed Mennonite farmer's chair, because of the way our pelvis rotates below the spine, we're bent forward about 20 degrees from standing alignment and the loads go up by a third. When we recline, the loads are cut in half . . . that's why we all like a recliner in the first place! Lying down is even better.

Many other researchers have built on these findings since then. There's a good body of work on spinal alignments — sitting versus standing versus slouching and so on. Biomechanics has looked at twisting, as a function of alignment of the collagen fibers in the outer part of the disc (the annulus). It's suggested that twisting will greatly amplify loads too.

Older readers may remember getting lectures about good posture in grade school, but being ramrod straight only matters when you're standing up! Sitting, let yourself recline (lean backwards) whenever you can. Certainly don't slouch forward unsupported a lot (gamers peering at their screens as they frantically manipulate their controllers?) because, again, the loads spike in that position . . . and if you are slouching, at least plunk your elbows down on the table to offload your back (effectively, supporting some of your body weight in front).

Anyone who does a lot of physical labor will have heard a lot about "lift with your legs, not your back . . ." It's *soooo* important, not so much because the leg muscles are bigger and stronger than the back muscles, but because keeping the spine erect while bending to lift drops the load on our discs so much.

So, Reader, here goes . . . here's how I've kept myself out of trouble. It's also what I teach and preach to my own real-world spine care and surgical patients every day about managing their spines to minimize overloads and to avoid injury.

MY LOW BACK ADVICE TO THE HEALTHY PATIENT (OR THOSE WITH MINOR SYMPTOMS)

Think about keeping straight, 24/7/365. That means being aware of keeping your spine straight whatever you are doing and not just when literally standing straight.

Heaven forbid I would bend over to tie my shoelaces or pick up something off the floor. After decades it's instinctive to me now: I purposefully "lock up" my arched low back and shorten by flexing my hips and knees simultaneously to lower my body towards the ground as in a squat, and I try to keep my back "locked up" as I rise back up. If I can, I'll grab whatever wall or piece of furniture is next to me for a little offloading boost on the way back up. If I find myself having to reach forward while down there, I always try to support myself on one outstretched arm while I use the other. When barefoot, I'm really good at picking stuff up with my toes too, to avoid bending over at all. (I know, TMI. Sorry.)

We get in trouble in the act of sitting. Going down to the chair, our "back" muscle system relaxes to let us bend forward, curving our spine until we hit the chair, and then we do the same thing on the way back up. *Bad bad bad.* When I'm going to sit, I back up against the chair until it brushes against the back of my calf, straighten up and piston straight down onto the leading edge of the chair. Only then do I shift backwards on the chair to recline against it. Older patients with stiff hips or knees should not be too proud to get elevated toilets in the home to minimize that dip; conventional toilets are usually even lower than a chair.

Getting up out of a chair is the same but worse. Heaven forbid one curls forward as in a sit-up to come forward from the reclined position. Biomechanical analysis of a sit-up shows it loads the spine at the upper safety limit of current Canadian work safety guidelines — and the spine bends forward into the risk position of flexion with the movement! Instead, I use my arms to push myself up straight, slide forward on the chair and then piston straight up in a reversal of my sitting-down maneuver.

Yes, it's true: a lot of commonly prescribed "back-strengthening" exercises, like sit-ups, are marginally unsafe due to their biomechanics. Interested readers might want to go to writings by my colleague Dr. Stuart McGill, who has been a world leader in this field for a long time. His book *Back Mechanic* is written for the patient. His others are written for medical professionals.

When sitting at a desk to do work, *recline recline recline*. Drop your chair down and tilt it back. Raise your computer screen up from the desk surface to encourage you to look up a bit to see it, which extends your neck and back. Try not to slouch when sitting, because that also spikes the load on your discs. Stay as erect as possible, and if you must sit for long periods of time, do one of two things: either actively arch up your back all the time (this feels a bit like sticking your bum out), or (this is best) slide forward on the chair so your pelvis can tilt forward a bit on the seat's front edge. That will arch your back protectively a bit.

One of those businesses that I've never seen help a back patient is ergonomics, which analyzes your workplace and modifies it for your comfort and safety — often with a very pricey special chair. They're all just cushions. I don't think they change your alignment one bit! The only piece of "ergo" research I've ever seen in my literature was an old article from China where seated factory workers were given stools that tilted forward and made them arch their backs a bit. Backache disability in that factory dropped like a stone.

I worry about gamers. I've actually treated a guy in his 30s who would spend all night cross-legged on the floor peering forward at his screens through the night, until one day he was unable to get up in the morning. His entire L5/S1 disc had been slowly pushed out of place. (He did OK after surgery.)

Your car's a big thing. Careful getting in and out if it's a smaller vehicle — a female patient described her maneuvering to me as being similar to what needs to be done when she's getting into the car wearing a miniskirt: hold the body straight, door open wide, one hand atop the door and the other on the rooftop edge, lower the body straight down towards the seat. In a bigger car, just the bend and reach to close the door can hurt. When my own back's acting up, I keep a snowbrush on the passenger seat and use it to hook the door closed.

Once in the car, recline your seat position a bit from the usual. Slide the seat forwards an inch or two, then tilt back to maintain your normal distance from the steering wheel. Makes a huge difference for me!

WHAT ABOUT STRENGTHENING YOUR BACK?

What's the point of all the focus in back care on strengthening, we might ask? Really it goes to biomechanics, posture and disc loads. When our back muscles relax with fatigue, our posture sags forward a bit, just like your elbow starts straightening out after a while if you try to hold a heavy dumbbell in your hand for too long. That leaning forward increases the pressure on the discs at the front of your spine and is asking for trouble. The point of back strengthening is to prevent that from happening.

Hmm, so what we *really* need in our spine is endurance, not strength. But I digress . . .

There's plenty of scientific and popular literature on what exercises to do and how well they all allegedly strengthen your back, often supported by pain scores and other "outcome measures." Maybe the pain was 5/10 or 6/10 before and 2 or 3 after, so these are the best exercises ever, right?

In fact, there's very little literature on whether any of them actually change where those patients are going to be a year or two or five or 10 later. That makes me very suspicious. My care plan always involves trying to find treatment that will help the patient feel so well relieved they'll be discharged from my practice permanently.

Early in my practice, I did what I was taught and what the literature supported: send people for active physical care up front to avoid surgery, and afterwards to get the best outcome. I got suspicious very fast because so many people came back from exercise therapy complaining that they were worse off for it, that it hurt.

Once again, I've had to remember that spines are different from the extremities. Forget "no pain, no gain" in spine care. Patients come to us for *relief* of their pain and other symptoms, not asking for more. There's nothing good about back pain.

After a decade or so, I started writing out long-winded pages of individualized therapy instructions for my people. Didn't work. The therapists never seemed to follow them.

After another decade, I bailed on it all. Instead, I pushed my people to take regular extended daily walks as a major component of their rehab, and I still do. (A brisk one-hour walk is usually about 5,000 steps on your iPhone or Fitbit.) A lot of people just won't do it, sadly. That's on them.

During all this time a consistent body of scientific literature emerged showing quite definitively that the single best exercise a person can do to strengthen their back is a simple thing called *planking*, which evolved from Pilates. For details, you can Google or YouTube it. I could explain it here but some visuals help a lot. Quite often, I actually get down on the floor and do a demo for my patients, and have them try it with me in the clinic!

As a spine patient (or somebody trying to avoid becoming one), stick to the basic planking technique where you're supported on both elbows and on your toes; there's no need to get fancy. There's no high-risk bending or twisting involved in doing it at all. I do worry about it being a floor exercise, however. For many of my patients, the gymnastics involved in getting down there and back up are an issue, so I have people do it in bed, ideally once in the morning before they make up the bedsheets and again in the evening before curling up for the night — that makes it an easy regular part of the day. But if you're healthy and doing this exercise for prevention, the floor should be fine.

I count slowly to myself while I'm holding a plank: one thousand, two thousand and so on. Most normal people seem to easily work up to planking for a minute or two, call it a count of a hundred — or use the timer on your phone. I started doing this exercise religiously when the gyms closed at the start of the COVID pandemic, and I could barely hold the planked position to a count of 15! It turns out I'm really good at planking: took all the COVID years but I'm regularly over 500 now.

Before COVID I'd come home from the OR exhausted and with a great big burning pain under my left shoulder blade, hit the couch after dinner and do nothing. I put it down to the intensity of all this complex spine surgery I was doing. Now I come home from the same ORs and I'm invigorated; my wife and I will often hit the gym or go for a long exercise walk on my OR day. It turns out I hadn't been coming home exhausted from operating; I was coming home exhausted because my scrawny atrophied back muscles weren't up to the job of supporting me upright for long enough to do the work! I still have my back pain; planking is no cure. But I have a lot less of it, and better comfort and stamina in the OR and at the gym than I've had in decades.

Oddly it seems one doesn't have to be religious about it. Having built my strength, I get lazy and "cheat" a lot, might not do a plank for several days when I'm busy. But when I go back to it my endurance is still there.

If everybody started walking and planking in their 30s, when our vitality and health generally start to drop off, I think I'd be largely out of a job.

MY NECK ADVICE TO THE HEALTHY PATIENT
(OR THOSE WITH MINOR SYMPTOMS)

It's been rare in my practice experience for me to see patients with just a sore neck. Virtually all the neck cases I see have widespread deterioration and neurological problems. So I can't propose as much tried-and-true prevention and management as I can for the low back patient, but the principles are the same and maybe a bit easier to understand through explanation.

Your head's as heavy as a bowling ball, around 10 pounds (or 5 kilograms). It's not balanced directly atop your shoulders but offset to the front a bit. That's why if we relax our neck muscles, the head falls forward. The muscles on the back of your neck are contracting all the time to prevent that, and the combination of pressure front and back puts a lot of load on the very small discs in the neck, which are only about a half inch in diameter.

So once again, *posture posture posture.* It just makes good common and biomechanical sense. And that's a big issue in today's world where we're peering down at screens of various sorts all day. Or reading, if you're me. So my best advice to the patient with a sore neck is to pay attention to all that. Elevate monitors and screens so you look forward (or even upwards a bit), not down. Keyboards, monitors and laptops can be supported on a thick book or any of a number of small platform devices commonly found at office supply stores.

Strengthening the neck I honestly know little about. I've never followed that literature much. For my patients, I suggest two simple things.

If planking, hold the neck straight and look down at the floor to keep your neck and back all in alignment and on one straight plane. For me, that's really hard. Shortly into my plank, my head is usually sagging downwards and I find myself staring at my belly; because my neck doesn't bother me or hurt regularly, I never pay attention to it.

For post-op neck patients, I often teach a simple isometric exercise, again an activity that doesn't involve a lot of bending and twisting. Standing or sitting erect and holding the head up straight, clasp your hands together behind the back of the head. Don't thrust the head backwards because that tends to roll the head upwards and doesn't work the support muscles well. Instead, imagine pulling the head forward with your hands and *resist* with the neck muscles while maintaining a level gaze. Hold the position for two or three seconds, relax, and repeat for a total of 10 or 12 reps. Ideally at least once every day if you're healthy and doing this for prevention, but I do bug my post-op patients to do it four times (meals and bedtime) until they're comfortable.

And that's as much on neck prevention as I can offer. Simple, but effective.

∫

It is a privilege to treat the surgical spine care patient, and a great joy to see the results of thorough and timely spine care. For a long time, I really didn't understand why spine care gets the bad rap that it does.

It took me years of practice, reading and learning to gain a real understanding of how the spine works and what surgical spine care can be. It took longer for me to realize that spine care gets its generally bad rap largely due to ignorance because the medical world doesn't teach much at all about spine care issues to the major medical audience, not to mention anybody else.

By sharing with you the reader here, I hope I have shown some of what surgical spine care really can be, lessened the fear and anxiety and confusion around it and assisted our patients to better outcomes.

Appendix
The Influencers

The impactful teachers who led me to writing this book.

D r. Joseph Miller was chief of orthopedics and director of the orthopedic training program at McGill when I trained there. Wonderful fellow, a classical English gentleman if a bit Canadianized. He was always proper and somewhat formal. If he was stressed, he'd never let it show, unlike most surgeons today. He taught me three things.

One was to strive for a deep understanding of the orthopedics I was learning. There wasn't much of an established teaching curriculum or time for teaching at McGill back then so as an alternative he'd advise us to read the original literature! You could do that at McGill in the era before the Internet and Google. Both the med school and the hospitals had wonderful old libraries that were quiet and smelled musty and had decades of old scientific journals and textbooks lying around. I spent a lot of time there trying to figure out what I wasn't being taught. It worked. I passed my boards my first time up.

Another was to try to improve on what we do. In the 1980s when I was training, total knee replacements (TKRs) were quite primitive and not very good. Joe worked with the Zimmer company (now Zimmer Biomet) developing several better devices, the most successful of which was Zimmer's first uncemented TKR called the *Miller-Galante knee* (Dr. Jorge Galante was apparently something of a metallurgist.) As trainee surgeons, we knew this was going on because Dr. Miller would sometimes talk about it in the OR but mostly it was rather hush-hush. I expect Zimmer didn't want us all to see what could become corporate secrets. "Uncle Joe" wasn't flashy and never bragged about the money that might be involved with all this. When he rarely did open up about his research, he spoke of it with genuine interest in designing joint replacements that would work better and last longer than they usually did at the time.

The third thing Joe taught me was the critical importance of family in a professional career. Broken families and old surgeons struggling to pay alimony to several ex-wives are still too common in my field. Joe's was solid. Dozens of times he'd say he'd travel to lecture anywhere and anytime without charging fees for his speaking engagements — but he insisted on first-class travel and accommodations for both him and his wife. Smart. I've modeled that in bringing my family along with me when traveling to lectures and meetings in many countries and never regretted a minute of it, despite the sad fact that (unlike Joe) it was all on my own dime.

Joe didn't want me to do spine; he likely thought I was nuts. There was very little adult spine surgery done at McGill at the time, and it didn't usually go well. When I asked for a reference letter to the program in Toronto, I almost made an enemy of him, I think. Sadly I never had a chance to thank him for all he gave me. He passed away shortly after I left Montreal.

∫

Dr. Stephen Ivor Esses. I got into Toronto for my fellowship as a bit of a squeaker, I think. Dr. John Kostuik was an established big name there and hosted two trainee fellows in spine surgery every year. Toronto had sent off one of their graduates, Dr. Stephen Esses, to specialize elsewhere, and when he returned I was appointed as his fellow, the second I believe. Pedicle screw technology was just emerging at the time and he was quite notorious for instrumenting over 50 patients with the things in his first year of practice when virtually nobody in Canada had ever done them. He taught me how to use these screws before there was any kind of a practice standard. We even did the things percutaneously (through the skin without a cut), which is very advanced even today. In the course of that, he also taught me to think about screw mechanics and bone biology a lot, and I wish more people did that. I believe there are fundamental shortcomings in much of screw fixation today that could likely be bettered if these things were taught, understood and practiced.

Most importantly Steve taught me to talk to patients, to work really hard in gathering their symptom history to understand what a given patient's problems and needs are before offering care. Do some Googling and you'll find an online video of him reaching out to patients that could set a standard for what every spine surgeon should aspire to do.

He also taught me to support my learners, to treat the students with some dignity and respect. Too many teachers don't. While working with him I was supporting my beautiful, wonderful, smart, fantastic wife and two-year-old twins on a base salary of $2,000 a month when rent was $1,600 for a musty old townhouse in downtown Toronto. We had just $400 left over to spend every month, which didn't buy a lot of diapers and groceries even then. Family helped us out a bit, but Steve took me and my wife out to dinner religiously once a month, keeping us fed and engaged with the world by giving us a little sanity break from the "rug rats," as he called them.

∫

Dr. John Kostuik ("JPK") was the Real Boss. A phenomenon. Pioneering surgeon in the field of spinal deformity decades before the rest of the world figured out the need, even before we had the implant technologies to do it properly. He ran the best-funded biomechanics research lab in the country at the time. But John wasn't respected much by the orthopedic community in Canada because he functioned at the most elite level of spine care in the world and Canada was then a place of country bumpkins who in the majority felt that pinched nerves were the only thing to treat surgically in spine care. When he would lecture and present cases in Canada, he was trash-talked all the time.

Honestly, I was rather afraid of him during my time in Toronto. He was The Great Man and I was only the Fellow of the New Kid (Dr. Esses). But I reached out as I could.

Dr. Kostuik taught me to track my data, to review my practice regularly to make sure people were doing as well as I expected they were and to try to do it a bit better every time — just as Drs. Miller and Esses did. I've never been the great scientist he is and so never approached his standard of having a nurse at his side collecting data from every patient, but I do what I can. Spine practice at McMaster isn't that kind of academic, and I've taken a lot of the same criticisms that JPK did in my time, but my patients' outcomes keep me on track, as his undoubtedly did.

Old-style Harrington spine fusions tended to straighten out the normal lumbar lordosis curvature, the hollow of your low back that lets you stand up straight. People were ending up with their spines solidly fused in positions that saw them pitched forward from the hips by 20, 30, sometimes 40 degrees or more. To correct this we did massive old-fashioned AP osteotomy operations, really two operations at once. We'd lie the patient on their side in the OR, one team (JPK and the senior residents) would open the belly to get to the front of the spine, and a second team (fellows and the interns) would open the back. We'd cut both the front and the back of the spine apart, realign it and screw it back together with whatever we could. Took all day, bled tons, put people into ICU on lots of narcotics. (Ironically, something very similar is a hot topic in MIS fusion practice today.)

But man did it work. True story: one day early in my training, a post-op patient of his showed up at clinic for suture removal on the wrong day. JPK was out of town, so I volunteered to take her sutures out. This well-dressed woman was in no obvious discomfort, and I expected to remove maybe a half dozen stitches from a little disc surgery wound. When she rolled up her shirt there was a 15-inch slash across her left belly and flank and another along the length of her low back. I was shocked! I took out dozens and dozens of surgical staples as she raved about how good she felt, how she was already using less painkiller than she had been before the surgery. Yeah, that's what good spine surgery can do for people. Orthopedics and most other disciplines can't touch that!

Dr. Kostuik really convinced me that was what I wanted to do for people when I'd grow up. I think I'm still growing.

∫

Dr. Hamilton Hall was an active Toronto orthopedic and spine surgeon when I trained. He's retired now but still functions as administrator of our Canadian Spine Society (spinecanada.ca). We never worked together, but early in my academic career, he encouraged me to apply for membership in the International Society for the Study of the Lumbar Spine (issls.org), then arguably the lead academic spine society anywhere. It's still up there. It has been a wonderful place to expand my thinking and work to understand how the spine works, what goes wrong with it and how we can best help the patient. Hamilton and I don't cross paths very often so we're not close and we likely disagree professionally a bit. I think I'm much more pro-surgery than he is. But that's OK; he greatly encouraged my "thinking forward." He also wrote a lot of spine books for public consumption, maybe that's not a bad idea . . .

∫

Constantina Nanos-Bednar, MA, RP, RMFT-SM, CSFT, AAMFT. OK sure, this is the woman I love and am married to. Not only has she been an unfailing supporter of my crazy enthusiasm for spine care, but she models the importance of professional dedication and the looking for small things that can lead to big differences. Dina is a national lead psychotherapist in the growing field of solution-focused brief therapy (SFBT), which teaches "go slow to be fast" and "slice it thin" (look for fine details). I've always taught surgical trainees to operate slowly for good outcome and few complications first; getting quick at it will come later. Maybe that's part of why I'm putting out this book at a late stage in my career. It's taken a very long time for me to be sure that I'm getting it right (not always, but most of the time).

Dina acquired all those letters, her expertise and her reputation only *after* being largely a single parent to our children who have a 10-year spread in age, so she illustrates the truth that even later in life one can learn widely and advance professionally to great heights. So, it's never too early to learn or too late to keep on learning. I learn something from every patient I see and every case I do.

Selected References

The expert spine care literature is enormous, and I will make no attempt to review it comprehensively here. I will only present some key literature. Some articles are classics and some are very recent definitive research. Most of these articles have their own extensive bibliographies attached, which can in turn take the interested reader into a great deal of detail.

I've added short notes to explain why I've included each article or grouping, or what the key point is.

THE BEST LITTLE SPINE BOOK EVER

Macnab's Backache: Fourth Edition, edited by David A. Wong and Ensor Transfeldt. Philadelphia: Lippincott Williams & Wilkins, 2007.

CHAPTER 1: JOHN THE ROOFER

Everything to know about median nerve anatomy and carpal tunnel syndrome.

Keith, Michael Warren, Victoria Masear, Kevin C. Chung, Peter C. Amadio, Michael Andary, Richard W. Barth, Kent Maupin, Brent Graham, William C. Watters 3rd, Charles M. Turkelson, Robert H. Haralson 3rd, Janet L. Wies and Richard McGowan. "American Academy of Orthopaedic Surgeons Clinical Practice Guideline on Diagnosis of Carpal Tunnel Syndrome." *Journal of Bone and Joint Surgery* 91, no. 1 (2009): 2478–2479. https://doi.org/10.2106/JBJS.I.00642.

Who was Sir William Osler?

Bliss, Michael. *William Osler: A Life in Medicine.* Toronto: University of Toronto Press, 1999.

Myelopathy versus Guillain-Barré syndrome — what should we worry about first?

Nouri, Aria, Lindsay Tetreault, Anoushka Singh, Spyridon K. Karadimas and Michael G. Fehlings. "Degenerative Cervical Myelopathy: Epidemiology, Genetics and Pathogenesis." *Spine* 40, no. 12 (June 2015): E675–E693. https://doi.org/10.1097/BRS.0000000000000913.

Alter, Milton. "The Epidemiology of Guillain-Barré Syndrome." *Annals of Neurology* 27, no. S1 (1990): S7–S12. https://doi.org/10.1002/ana.410270704.

And just how long have we known that myelopathy is a very common problem?

Nurick, S. "The Natural History and the Results of Surgical Treatment of the Spinal Cord Disorder Associated with Cervical Spondylosis." *Brain* 95, no. 1 (1972): 101–108. https://doi.org/10.1093/brain/95.1.101.

CSM: How common is it? How long are people symptomatic before diagnosis? How should it be managed and does the surgery work?

Fehlings, Michael G., Jefferson R. Wilson, Branko Kopjar, Sangwook Tim Yoon, Paul M. Arnold, Eric M. Massicotte, Alexander R. Vaccaro, Darrel S. Brodke, Christopher I. Shaffrey, Justin S. Smith, et al. "Efficacy and Safety of Surgical Decompression in Patients with Cervical Spondylotic Myelopathy. Results of the AO Spine North America Prospective Multi-Center Study." *Journal of Bone and Joint Surgery* 95, no. 18 (September 2013): 1651–1658. https://doi.org/10.2106/JBJS.L.00589.

Fehlings, Michael G., Ahmed Ibrahim, Lindsay Tetreault, Vincenzo Albanese, Manuel Alvarado, Paul Arnold, Giuseppe Barbagallo, Ronald Bartels, Ciaran Bolger, Helton Defino, et al. "A Global Perspective on the Outcomes of Surgical Decompression in Patients with Cervical Spondylotic Myelopathy. Results from the Prospective Multicenter AO Spine International Study on 479 Patients." *Spine* 40, no. 7 (2015): 1322–1328. https://doi.org/10.1097/BRS.0000000000000988.

CHAPTER 2: HORACE THE DENTIST

How thorough is the average doctor's musculoskeletal education?

Goff, Ian, Elspeth Mary Wise, David Coady and David Walker. "Musculoskeletal Training: Are GP Trainees Exposed to the Right Case Mix for Independent Practice?" *Clinical Rheumatology* 35, no. 2 (February 2016): 507–511. https://doi.org/10.1007/s10067-014-2767-z.

Murphy, Robert F., Dawn M. LaPorte and Veronica M.R. Wadey. "Current Concepts Review. Musculoskeletal Education in Medical School: Deficits in Knowledge and Strategies for Improvement." *Journal of Bone and Joint Surgery* 96, no. 23 (December 2014): 2009–2014. https://doi.org/10.2106/JBJS.N.00354.

What are "red flags"?

Premkumar, Ajay, William Godfrey, Michael B. Gottschalk and Scott D. Boden. "Red Flags for Low Back Pain Are Not Always Really Red: A Prospective Evaluation of the Clinical Utility of Commonly Used Screening Questions for Low Back Pain." *Journal of Bone and Joint Surgery* 100, no. 5 (March 2018): 368–74. https://doi.org/10.2106/JBJS.17.00134.

Wong, Hee-Kit. "Should We Still Use Red Flags in the Diagnosis of Low Back Pain?: Commentary on an Article by Ajay Premkumar, MD, MPH, et al.: 'Red Flags for Low Back Pain Are Not Always Really Red. A Prospective Evaluation of the Clinical Utility of Commonly Used Screening Questions for Low Back Pain.'" *Journal of Bone and Joint Surgery* 100, no. 5 (March 2018): e31. https://doi.org/10.2106/JBJS.17.01391.

What are all these spinal infections?

Brody, Barrett D., Tyler J. Jenkins, Joseph Maslak, Wellington K. Hsu and Alpesh A. Patel. "Vertebral Osteomyelitis and Spinal Epidural Abscess: An Evidence-Based Review." *Journal of Spinal Disorders and Technique* 28, no. 6 (July 2015): E316–E327. https://doi.org/10.1097/BSD.0000000000000294.

CHAPTER 3: FRANK THE TRUCKER

What are Waddell's signs, and what are they all about?

Waddell, Gordon, John A. McCulloch, E. Kummel and Robert M. Venner. "Nonorganic Physical Signs in Low-Back Pain." *Spine* 5, no. 2 (March 1980): 117–125. https://doi.org/10.1097/00007632-198003000-00005.

Waddell, Gordon, Mansel Aylward and Philip Sawney. *Back Pain, Incapacity of Work and Social Security Benefits: An International*

Literary Review and Analysis. London: Royal Society of Medicine Press, 2002.

The pain centralization score is a thing!

Neblett, Randy, Howard Cohen, YunHee Choi, Meredith M. Hartzell, Mark Williams, Tom G. Mayer and Robert J. Gatchel. "The Central Sensitization Inventory (CSI): Establishing Clinically Significant Values for Identifying Central Sensitivity Syndromes in an Outpatient Chronic Pain Sample." *Journal of Pain* 14, no. 5 (May 2013): 438–445. https://doi.org/10.1016/j.jpain.2012.11.012.

The pain catastrophizing score is a thing too!

Sullivan, M.J.L., S. Bishop and J. Pivik. "The Pain Catastrophizing Scale: Development and Validation." *Psychological Assessment* 7, no. 4 (1995): 524–532. https://doi.org/10.1037/1040-3590.7.4.524.

A bit about how your spine actually works.

Gracovetshy, S., H.F. Farfan and C. Lamy. "The Mechanism of the Lumbar Spine." *Spine* 6, no. 3 (1981): 249–262. https://doi.org/10.1097/00007632-198105000-00007.

Here's something on that kinetic thing around disc malfunction in the "bearing" function, and why "walking hands up the thighs" actually works for some people.

Gertzbein, S.D., J Seligman, R. Holtby, K.W. Chan, N. Ogston, A. Kapasouri and M. Tile. "Centrode Characteristics of the Lumbar Spine as a Function of Segmental Instability." *Clinical Orthopaedics and Related Research* 208 (July 1988): 48–51.

Dickey, James P., Michael R. Pierrynowski, Drew A. Bednar and Simon X. Yang. "Relationship between Pain and Vertebral Motion in Chronic Low-Back Pain Subjects." *Clinical Biomechanics* 17, no. 5 (June 2002): 345–352. https://doi.org/10.1016/s0268-0033(02)00032-3.

What is the discogram and why use it?

Derby, Richard, Mark W. Howard, Joseph M. Grant, John J. Lettice, P.K. Van Peteghem and Deaglán P. Ryan. "The Ability of Pressure-Controlled Discography to Predict Surgical and Nonsurgical Outcomes." *Spine* 24, no. 4 (February 1999): 364–372.

Guyer, Richard D. and Donna D. Ohnmeiss. "NASS: Lumbar Discography." *The Spine Journal* S3 (May 2003): S11–S27. https://doi.org/10.1016/s1529-9430(02)00563-6.

On sagittal balance.

Mehta, Vivek A., Anubhav Amin, Ibrahim Omeis, Ziya L. Gokaslan and Oren N. Gottfried. "Implications of Spinopelvic Alignment for the Spine Surgeon." *Neurosurgery* 70, no. 3 (March 2012): 707–721. https://doi.org/10.1227/NEU.0b013e31823262ea.

Diebo, Bassel G., Neil V. Shah, Oheneba Boachie-Adjei, Feng Zhu, Dominique A. Rothenfluh, Carl B. Paulino, Frank J. Schwab and Virginie Lafage. "Adult Spinal Deformity." *Lancet* 394 (July 2019): 160–172. https://doi.org/10.1016/S0140-6736(19)31125-0.

CHAPTER 4: MIKE THE MANAGER

All about the sacroiliac joint, and a lot of low-probability data.

Glaser, J. "Chapter 20: Sacroiliac Joint Dysfunction." In *Orthopedic Knowledge Update: Spine 5*, edited by Eeric Truumees and Heidi Prather, 283–292. Rosemont, Illinois: American Academy of Orthopaedic Surgeons, 2017.

Kosukegawa, Ima, Mitsunori Yoshimoto, Satoshi Isogai, Shinsuke Nonaka and Toshihiko Yamashita. "Piriformis Syndrome Resulting from a Rare Anatomic Variation." *Spine* 31, no. 18 (August 2006): E664–E666. https://www.nejm.org/doi/pdf/10.1056/NEJM 193408022110506.

Classics on disc hernia, and how it usually gets better without help.

Mixter, William Jason, and Joseph S. Barr. "Rupture of the Intervertebral Disc with Involvement of the Spinal Canal." *New England Journal of Medicine* 210 (August 1934): 205–210.

Komori, Hiromichi, Kenichi Shinomiya, Osamu Nakai, Isakichi Yamaura, Syuichi Takeda and Kohtaro Furuya. "The Natural History of Herniated Nucleus Pulposus with Radiculopathy." *Spine* 21, no. 2 (1996): 225–229.

Postacchini, Fran. "Results of Surgery Compared with Conservative Management for Lumbar Disc Herniations." *Spine* 21, no. 11 (June 1996): 1383–1387. https://doi.org/10.1097/00007632 -199606010-00023.

Disc surgery really is commonly day surgery, MIS or not!

Bednar, Drew A. "Analysis of Factors Affecting Successful Discharge in Patients Undergoing Lumbar Discectomy for Sciatica Performed on a Day-Surgical Basis: A Prospective Study of Sequential Cohorts." *Journal of Spinal Disorders and Technique* 12, no. 5 (October 1999): 359–362.

Best, Matthew J., Leonard T. Buller and Frank J. Eismont. "National Trends in Ambulatory Surgery for Intervertebral Disc Disorders and Spinal Stenosis: A 12-Year Analysis of the National Surveys of Ambulatory Surgery." *Spine* 40, no. 21 (November 2015): 1703–1711. https://doi.org/10.1097/BRS.0000000000001109.

Arshi, Armin, Howard Y. Park, Gideon W. Blumstein, Christopher Wang, Zorica Buser, Jeffrey C. Wang, Arya N. Shamie and Don Y. Park. "Outpatient Posterior Lumbar Fusion: A Population-Based Analysis of Trends and Complication Rates." *Spine* 43, no. 22 (2018): 1559–1565. https://doi.org/10.1097/BRS .0000000000002664.

CHAPTER 5: MARY THE PSW

What is internal medicine?

OK, this isn't a reference from the literature but an explanation. Internal medicine is that discipline best dedicated to "making the diagnosis" of a case and treating optimally, generally with medicines rather than injections or surgery. These are the doctors who are supposed to know everything there is to know about what goes on inside of us, hence the "internal" moniker. It's the foundation of a specialty medical career; generally you have to be certified in internal medicine before even starting to train say in cardiology or neurology or whatever. Remember the TV series *House*, about a challenged physician genius who could always figure out what was wrong when nobody else could? Dr. House was an internist.

What's a differential diagnosis?

This is the list of what-could-it-be's that the internist composes after interviewing and examining the patient. Ideally, the most common or likely problems are at the top of the list and the rarer options are lower down.

What's a diagnostic workup?

This is the menu of tests proposed to help us make the diagnosis as quickly and efficiently as possible.

What is a bedsore?

These are also called *decubitus ulcers*. It takes very little pressure to block the flow of blood to our tissues. Pinch your thumbnail up against the tip of another finger and that finger turns white because blood flow has been occluded — you don't have to push hard to do that. Keep it pinched for too long and the fingertip will start to hurt; later it turns red and ultimately it might die, turn black and fall off. This is a risk anywhere there's the pressure of our body up against the external environment. It's why we fidget in a seat or toss and turn in bed — we're protecting ourselves from these bedsores! Here's a nice readable review article:

Bluestein, D., A Javaheri. "Pressure Ulcers: Prevention, Evaluation, and Management." *American Family Physician* 78, no. 10 (2008): 1186–1194.

Spine isn't a big item in the medical school curriculum.

McMaster's med school is called the Michael G. DeGroote School of Medicine. Google us and hunt around through the curriculum on the website; it's openly available there, as are those of most medical schools. I can't even find the word *spine* in there. I am not the only person concerned about this.

Ye, Albert C., Orrin Franko and Charles S. Day. "Impact of Clinical Electives and Residency Interest on Medical Students' Education in Musculoskeletal Medicine." *Journal of Bone and Joint Surgery* 90, no. 2 (2008): 307–315. https://doi.org/10.2106/JBJS.G.00472.

Murphy, Robert F., Dawn M. LaPorte and Veronica M.R. Wadey. "Current Concepts Review. Musculoskeletal Education in Medical School: Deficits in Knowledge and Strategies for Improvement." *Journal of Bone and Joint Surgery* 96, no. 23 (December 2014): 2009–2014. https://doi.org/10.2106/JBJS.N.00354.

Goff, Ian, Elspeth Mary Wise, David Coady and David Walker. "Musculoskeletal Training: Are GP Trainees Exposed to the Right Case Mix for Independent Practice?" *Clinical Rheumatology* 35, no. 2 (February 2016): 507–511. https://doi.org/10.1007/s10067-014-2767-z.

On nerve fiber diameters, and more.

Histology is the study of tissue structure at the microscopic level. My histology textbooks are really old so here's a great link: https://www.nysora.com/foundations-of-regional-anesthesia/anatomy/histology-peripheral-nerves-light-microscopy/.

How do we best take a spine patient's low back X-rays?

Cho, C.H. and R.M. Kurtz "Chapter 6: Spine Imaging." In *Orthopedic Knowledge Update: Spine 5*, edited by Eeric Truumees and

Heidi Prather, 73–86. Rosemont, Illinois: American Academy of Orthopedic Surgeons, 2017.

North American Spine Society. "Evidence-Based Clinical Guidelines for Multidisciplinary Spine Care: Diagnosis and Treatment of Degenerative Lumbar Spondylolisthesis." Revised 2014. https://www.spine.org/Portals/O/Documents/ResearchClinicalCare/Guidelines/Spondylolisthesis.pdf.

CHAPTER 6: LARRY THE LAWYER

How commonly does cancer go to the spine and does nonoperative care help?

Kumar, Abhishek, Michael H. Weber, Ziya Gokaslan, Jean-Paul Wolinsky, Meic Schmidt, Laurence Rhines, Michael G. Fehlings, Ilya Laufer, Daniel M. Sciubba, Michelle J. Clarke, Narayan Sundaresan, Jorrit-Jan Verlaan, Arjun Sahgal, Dean Chou and Charles G. Fisher. "Metastatic Spinal Cord Compression and Steroid Treatment: A Systematic Review." *Clinical Spine Surgery* 30 (2017): 156–163.

How well can people paralyzed by cancer in the spine do with surgery?

Patchell, Roy A., Phillip A. Tibbs, William F. Regine, Richard Payne, Stephen Saris, Richard J. Kryscio, Mohammed Mohiuddin and Byron Young. "Direct Decompressive Surgical Resection in the Treatment of Spinal Cord Compression Caused by Metastatic Cancer: A Randomised Trial." *Lancet* 366 (2005): 643–648. https://doi.org/10.1016/S0140-6736(05)66954-1.

How badly off you are when the problem is recognized best determines your chances of neurological recovery.

Laufer, Ilya, Scott L. Zuckerman, Justin E. Bird, Mark H. Bilsky, Áron Lazáry, Nasir A. Quraishi, Michael G. Fehlings, Daniel M.

Sciubba, John H. Shin, Addisu Mesfin, Arjun Sahgal and Charles G. Fisher. "Predicting Neurologic Recovery after Surgery in Patients with Deficits Secondary to Metastatic Epidural Spinal Cord Compression." *Spine* 41, no. 20S (2016): S224–S230. https://doi.org/10.1097/BRS.0000000000001827.

CHAPTER 7: SAMANTHA'S SORE FOOT

Can people close to paralyzed from spinal cord compression really recover, and if so, how fast and how well?

Kopjar, Branko, Parker E. Bohm, Joshua H. Arnold, Michael G. Fehlings, Lindsay A. Tetreault and Paul M. Arnold. "Outcomes of Surgical Decompression in Patients with Very Severe Degenerative Cervical Myelopathy." *Spine* 43, no. 16 (August 2018): 1102–1109. https://doi.org/10.1097/BRS.0000000000002602.

The role of parallel bars or walking rails in neurorehabilitation — these are nothing new!

Jin, Zlrenxing and Howard Jay Chizeck. "Instrumented Parallel Bars for Three-Dimensional Force Measurement." *Journal of Rehabilitation Research* 29, no. 2 (1992): 31–38. https://doi.org/10.1682/jrrd.1992.04.0031.

Visintin, M. and H. Barbeau. "The Effects of Parallel Bars, Body Weight Support and Speed on the Modulation of the Locomotor Pattern of Spastic Paretic Gait: A Preliminary Communication." *Spinal Cord* 32 (1994): 540–553. https://doi.org/10.1038/sc.1994.86.

Dobkin, Bruce H. and Andrew Dorsch. "New Evidence for Therapies in Stroke Rehabilitation." *Current Atherosclerosis Reports* 15, no. 6 (June 2013): 331.

Can pain really be absent in severe neurological compressions?

There are several subcategories within this major topic.

Of the spinal cord in the neck/CSM.

Bednarik, Josef, Zdenek Kadanka, Ladislav Dusek, Oldrich
Novotny, Dagmar Surelova, Igor Urbanek and Boleslav
Prokes. "Presymptomatic Spondylotic Cervical Cord
Compression." *Spine* 29, no. 20 (October 2004): 2260–2269.
https://doi.org/10.1097/01.brs.0000142434.02579.84.

In lumbar spinal stenosis.

Hall, Stephan, John D. Bartleson, Burton M. Onofrio, Hillier L.
Baker Jr., Haruo Okazaki and J. Desmond O'Duffy. "Lumbar
Spinal Stenosis. Clinical Features, Diagnostic Procedures and
Results of Surgical Treatment in 68 Patients." *Annals of Internal
Medicine* 103, no. 2 (1985): 271–275. https://doi.org/10.7326/0003
-4819-103-2-271.

Katz, Jeffrey N., Marianne Dalgas, Gerold Stucki, Nathaniel
P. Katz, James Bayley, Anne H. Fossel, Lily C. Chang and
Stephen J. Lipson. "Degenerative Lumbar Spinal Stenosis.
Diagnostic Value of the History and Physical Examination."
Arthritis and Rheumatology 38, no. 9 (1995): 1236–1241. https://
doi.org/10.1002/art.1780380910.

Germon, Timothy J. and Jeremy C. Hobart. "Definitions,
Diagnosis, and Decompression in Spinal Surgery: Problems
and Solution," *Spine* 15, no. 3 (2015): S5–S8. https://doi.org
/10.1016/j.spinee.2014.12.147.

In this British review article almost *1 in 10* patients had no
major pain!

In disc hernia and the sciatic syndromes.

Sciatica is all about leg (and bum!) pain. The actual low back
often doesn't hurt at all, and disc hernias can be discovered in
people entirely without symptoms!

Boden, S. D., D.O. Davis, T.S. Dina, N.J. Patronas and S.W. Wiesel. "Abnormal Magnetic Resonance Scans of the Lumbar Spine in Asymptomatic Subjects: A Prospective Investigation." *Journal of Bone and Joint Surgery* 72, no. 3 (March 1990): 403–408.

How accurate — or not — is the physical exam for sciatica?

Rebain, Richard, G. David Baxter and Suzanne McDonough. "A Systematic Review of the Passive Straight Leg Raising Test as a Diagnostic Aid for Low Back Pain (1989 to 2000)." *Spine* 27, no. 17 (September 2002): E388–E395. https://doi.org/10.1097/00007632 -200209010-00025.

De Luigi, Arthur J. and Kevin F. Fitzpatrick. "Physical Examination in Radiculopathy." *Physical Medicine and Rehabilitation Clinics of North America* 22, no. 1 (February 2011): 7–40. https://doi.org /10.1016/j.pmr.2010.10.003.

Electrophysiological testing isn't perfectly accurate either.

Dillingham, Timothy R. "Evaluating the Patient with Suspected Radiculopathy." *Physical Medicine and Rehabilitation* 5, no. 5S (May 2013): S41–49. https://doi.org/10.1016/j.pmrj.2013.03.015.

What are — or aren't — the implications of a spinal fluid leak, particularly in the neck?

O'Neill, K.R., Michael G. Fehlings, Thomas E. Mroz, Zachary A. Smith, Wellington K. Hsu, Adam S. Kanter, Michael P. Steinmetz, Paul M. Arnold, V. Mummaneni and Dean Chou. "A Multicenter Study of the Presentation, Treatment, and Outcomes of Cervical Dural Tears." *Global Spine Journal* 7, no. 1S (April 2017): 58S–63S. https://doi.org/10.1177/2192568216688186.

How common are hip and knee arthritis in an elderly population?

This population survey from Spain tells us both that hip and knee arthritis are very common and most of it doesn't warrant any surgery.

Quintana, José M., Inmaculada Arostegui, Antonio Escobar, Jesus Azkarate, J. Ignacio Goenaga and Iratxe Lafuente. "Prevalence of Knee and Hip Osteoarthritis and the Appropriateness of Joint Replacement in an Older Population." *Arch Intern Med.* 168, no. 14 (July 2008): 1576–1584. https://doi.org/10.1001 /archinte.168.14.1576.

What's the best anesthesia for total joint replacement?

Paziuk, Taylor M., Andrew J. Luzzi, Andrew N. Fleischman, Karan Goswami, Eric S. Schwenk, Eric A. Levicoff and Javad Parvizi. "General vs Spinal Anesthesia for Total Joint Arthroplasty: A Single-Institution Observational Review." *Journal of Arthoplasty* 35, no. 4 (April 2020): 955–959. https://doi.org/10.1016/j.arth .2019.11.019.

Turnbull, Zachary A., Dahniel Sastow, Gregory P. Giambrone and Tiffany Tedore. "Anesthesia for the Patient Undergoing Total Knee Replacement: Current Status and Future Prospects." *Local and Regional Anesthesiology* 10 (2017): 1–7. https://doi.org/10.2147 /LRA.S101373.

What is this new "anterior approach" for hip replacement all about?

Kyriakopoulos, Georgios, Lazaros Poultsides and Panayiotis Christofilopoulos. "Total Hip Arthroplasty Through an Anterior Approach: The Pros and Cons." *European Federation of National Associations of Orthopedics and Traumatology Open Reviews* 3, no. 11 (November 2018): 574–583. https://doi.org/10.1302/2058-5241.3 .180023.

Day surgery for disc hernia is nothing new, even with old-fashioned "open" technique.

Bednar, Drew A. "Analysis of Factors Affecting Successful Discharge in Patients Undergoing Lumbar Discectomy for Sciatica Performed on a Day-Surgical Basis: A Prospective Study of Sequential Cohorts." *Journal of Spinal Disorders and Techniques* 12, no. 5 (1999): 359–362.

Pre-op screening for optimization of cardiac risk in spine patients really is a thing.

Carabini, Louanne M., Carine Zeeni, Natalie C. Moreland, Robert W. Gould, Laura B. Hemmer, John F. Bebawy, Tyler R. Koski, Jamal McClendon Jr., Antoun Koht and Dhanesh K. Gupta. "Predicting Major Adverse Cardiac Events in Spine Fusion Patients: Is the Revised Cardiac Risk Index Sufficient?" *Spine* 39, no. 17 (August 2014): 1441–1448. https://doi.org/10.1097/BRS .0000000000000405.

What is the LAD: the left anterior descending coronary artery?

The biggest artery bringing blood to the heart. Cardiologists call it the "widow maker." Here's a recent article looking at best treatment options:

Codner, Pablo, Majdi Saada, Orazbek Sakhov, Jawed Polad, Fazila Tun-Nesa Malik, Shahzad Munir, Mamas Mamas, Jim Crowley, Jacques Monsegu, Luis Perez, Sasko Kedev, David Austin and Ariel Roguin. "Proximal Left Anterior Descending Artery Treatment Using a Bioresorbable Polymer Coating Sirolimus-Eluting Stent: Real-World Outcomes from the Multicenter Prospective e-Ultimaster Registry." *Journal of the American Heart Association* 8, no. 23 (December 2019): e013786. https://doi.org /10.1161/JAHA.119.013786.

Self-directed exercise after spine surgery is just as good as formal physio.

Fernandez, Matt, Jan Hartvigsen, Manuela L. Ferreira, Kathryn M. Refshauge, Aryane F. Machado, Ítalo R. Lemes, Chris G. Maher and Paulo H. Ferreira. "Advice to Stay Active or Structured Exercise in the Management of Sciatica: A Systematic Review and Meta-analysis." *Spine* 40, no. 18 (September 2015): 1457–1466. https://doi.org/10.1097/BRS.0000000000001036.

CHAPTER 9: BRIAN THE TEENAGER SKIPPING SCHOOL

Radiation exposure from CT scans can be dangerous.

Vaishnav, Avani S., Robert K. Merrill, Harvinder Sandhu, Steven J. McAnany, Sravisht Iyer, Catherine Himo Gang, Todd J. Albert and Sheeraz A. Qureshi. "A Review of Techniques, Time Demand, Radiation Exposure, and Outcomes of Skin-Anchored Intraoperative 3D Navigation in Minimally Invasive Lumbar Spinal Surgery." *Spine* 45, no. 8 (April 2020): E465–E476. https://doi.org/10.1097/BRS.0000000000003310.

Lin, Eugene C. "Radiation Risk from Medical Imaging." *Mayo Clinic Proceedings* 83, no. 12 (2010): 1142–1146. https://doi.org/10.4065/mcp.2010.0260.

Surgery is not generally very helpful for nonspecific low back pain.

Ibrahim, T., I. M. Tleyjeh and O. Gabbar. "Surgical Versus Non-surgical Treatment of Chronic Low Back Pain: A Meta-analysis of Randomised Trials." *International Orthopedics* 32, no. 1 (2008): 107–113.

Bydon, Mohamad, Rafael De la Garza-Ramos, Mohamed Macki, Abdul Baker, Aaron K. Gokaslan and Ali Bydon. "Lumbar Fusion Versus Non-operative Management for Treatment of Discogenic Low Back Pain: A Systematic Review and Meta-analysis of

Randomized Control Trials." *Journal of Spinal Disorders and Techniques* 27, no. 5 (2014): 297–304. https://doi.org/10.1097/BSD .0000000000000072.

Back pain is a common early symptom of lumbar disc hernia.

Aleem, I.S., R.D. Patel and A. Nassr. "Chapter 17: Lumbar Disc Herniations." In *Orthopedic Knowledge Update: Spine 5*, edited by Eeric Truumees and Heidi Prather, 243–251. Rosemont, Illinois: American Academy of Orthopaedic Surgeons, 2017.

Being unable to pee makes disc hernia an emergency.

Qureshi, Assad and Philip Sell. "Acute Cauda Equina Syndrome Caused by a Disc Herniation: Is Emergency Surgery the Correct Option? Surgical Decompression Remains the Standard of Care." *Spine* 40, no. 9 (2015): 639–641. https://doi.org/10.1007/s00586 -007-0491-y.

Most people recover quickly from an acute back pain episode — and it often comes back!

Stanton, Tasha R., Nicholas Henschke, Chris G. Maher, Kathryn M. Refshauge, Jane Latimer and James H. McAuley. "After an Episode of Acute Low Back Pain, Recurrence Is Unpredictable and Not as Common as Previously Thought." *Spine* 33, no. 26 (2008): 2923–2928. https://doi.org/10.1097/BRS.0b013e31818a3167.

Flexion gives relief of spinal stenosis symptoms by opening the spinal canal internally.

Alvarez, J.A. and R.H. Hardy. "Lumbar Spine Stenosis: A Common Cause of Back and Leg Pain." *American Family Physician* 57, no. 8 (1998): 1825–1834.

This is a simply fantastic and very well-illustrated review article on spinal stenosis that anybody like me would have been proud to write; it would be a great addition to the med school reading list.

What are secondary gains?

Docs are, I think, in the majority simplistic in their approach to this issue. In orthopedics, we off-the-record learn "he's just a bum faking backache to get off work (there's the primary gain) and a life of free money from the compensation board (that's the secondary gain)." But it's a lot more complex than that — I could almost write a book about it from my own practice experiences!

Here's yet another old-but-great review article that's very clear, well written and informative. Not a hot core-medical topic today so most recent pubs are blogs and links to the sites of behavioural therapists of various sorts, and often those are great too. I very much liked one from psychologist Arielle Schwartz, for what it's worth.

Fishbain, David A. "Secondary Gain Concept. Definition Problems and Its Abuse in Medical Practice." *American Psychiatric Society Journal* 3, no. 4 (1994): 264–273. https://doi.org/10.1016/S1058-9139 (05)80274-8.

van Egmond, J. J. "Multiple Meanings of Secondary Gain." *American Journal of Psychoanalysis* 63 (2003): 137–147. https://doi.org/10.1023 /a:1024027131335.

Acute disabling back pain in the majority resolves all by itself in a month or two.

There's a ton of literature on this out there, here's a great classic:

Bergquist-Ullmanand, Marianne and Ulf Larsson. "Acute Low Back Pain in Industry." *Acta Orthopedica Scandinavica* 170, S (1977): 1–117.

A bit about lumbar disc — and disc injury — mechanics.

Biomechanics gets complex really fast, but like all mechanics in its essence, it's simple. I generally like Margareta Nordin's classic book *Basic Biomechanics of the Musculoskeletal System*, the spine section there is terrific, but my best-ever single read would unquestionably be . . .

"Chapter 1. Musculoskeletal Anatomy, Neuroanatomy and Biomechanics of the Lumbar Spine." In *Macnab's Backache: Fourth Edition*, edited by David A. Wong and Ensor Transfeldt. Philadelphia: Lippincott Williams & Wilkins, 2007.

. . . and these peer-reviewed articles are pretty good too.

Veres, Samuel P., Peter A. Robertson and Neil D. Broom "ISSLS Prize Winner: How Loading Rate Influences Disc Failure Mechanics: A Microstructural Assessment of Internal Disruption." *Spine* 35, no. 21 (October 2010): 1897–1908. https://doi.org/10.1097/BRS.0b013e3181d9b69e.

Desmoulin, Geoffrey Thor, Vikram Pradhan and Theodore Edgar Milner. "Literature Review. Mechanical Aspects of Intervertebral Disc Injury and Implications on Biomechanics." *Spine* 45, no. 8 (April 2020): E457–E464. https://doi.org/10.1097/BRS.0000000000003291.

What is a black disc?

This is textbook stuff not published on commonly today. In certain MRI image sequences (called *T2-weighted*), which surgeons generally prefer, things that are fluid look white or light grey. As a disc starts to wear out, it loses water content and turns black, often while X-rays may still look perfectly normal. This is an early abnormality that is both very common and in the majority asymptomatic.

Boden, S.D., P.R. McCowin, D.O. Davis, T.S. Dina, A.S. Mark and S.W. Wiesel. "Abnormal Magnetic Resonance Scans of the Lumbar Spine in Asymptomatic Subjects." *Journal of Bone and Joint Surgery* 72, no. 3 (March 1990): 403–408.

Pfirrmann, Christian W.A., Alexander Metzdorf, Marco Zanetti, Juerg Hodler and Norbert Boos. "Magnetic Resonance Classification of Lumbar Intervertebral Disc Degeneration." *Spine* 26, no. 17 (September 2001): 1873–1878.

Bone marrow MRI abnormalities around a degenerated disc?

Modic, M.T., P.M. Steinberg, J.S. Ross, T.J. Masaryk and J.R. Carter. "Degenerative Disc Disease: Assessment of Changes in Vertebral Bone Marrow with MR Imaging." *Radiology* 166 (January 1988): 193–199. https://doi.org/10.1148/radiology.166.1.3336678.

Get your low back X-rays done with the patient standing up!

Cho, C.H. and R.M. Kurtz. "Chapter 6. Spine Imaging." In *Orthopedic Knowledge Update: Spine 5*, edited by Eeric Truumees and Heidi Prather, 73–86. Rosemont, Illinois: American Academy of Orthopaedic Surgeons, 2017.

North American Spine Society. "Evidence-Based Clinical Guidelines for Multidisciplinary Spine Care: Diagnosis and Treatment of Degenerative Lumbar Spondylolisthesis." Revised 2014. https:// www.spine.org/Portals/O/Documents/ResearchClinicalCare /Guidelines/Spondylolisthesis.pdf.

A bit about disc replacement, or disc arthroplasty.

Delamarter, Rick, Jack E. Zigler, Richard A. Balderston, Frank P. Cammisa, Jeffrey A. Goldstein and Jeffrey M. Spivak. "Prospective, Randomized Multicenter FDA IDE Study of the Prodisc-L Total Disc Replacement Compared with Circumferential Arthrodesis for the Treatment of Two-Level Lumbar Degenerative Disc Disease: Results at Twenty-Four Months." *Journal of Bone and Joint Surgery* 93, no. 8 (April 2011): 705–715. https://doi.org/10.2106/JBJS.I.00680.

Zigler, Jack E. and Rolando Garcia. "International Society for the Advancement of Spine Surgery Policy Statement: Lumbar Artificial Disc." *International Journal of Spine Surgery* 9 (March 2015): 7. https://doi.org/10.14444/2007.

What are the odds of another disc wearing out after successful surgery?

There is a big literature here again but it boils down to what I call the "Hilibrand number," roughly 3 percent per year of life.

Hilibrand, Alan S., Gregory Carlson, Mark A. Palumbo and Paul K. Jones. "Radiculopathy and Myelopathy at Segments Adjacent to the Site of a Previous Anterior Cervical Arthrodesis." *Journal of Bone and Joint Surgery* 81, no. 4 (1999): 519–528.

What is spinal instability?

Our spine joints can obviously move a bit. Abnormal motion is considered a bad thing, a sign of "instability" that might explain symptoms and warrant treatment. Two Canadians, William Kirkaldy-Willis and Harry Farfan, pioneered the concept of instability. Early on there was a large body of research devoted to defining the normal limits of motion. I learned, for example, that in the low back a wiggle of more than 3.5 millimeters or a bend of more than 11 degrees was abnormal — and saw surgeons take rulers and protractors to the X-rays to make treatment decisions! Not good. Our best definition today actually comes from one of the great gurus of hard-core biomechanics, Manohar Panjabi, one of whose articles I present you below. It's in his classic textbook, *Clinical Biomechanics of the Spine*, and it's in English. It's the basic "inability of the spine to support physiological loads without progressive deformity, neurological compression or uncontrolled pain."

Kirkaldy-Willis, William H. and Harry Farfan. "Instability of the Lumbar Spine." *Clinical Orthopedics and Related Research* 1 (1982): 110–123.

Panjabi, M.M., T.R. Oxland, I. Yamamoto and J.J. Crisco. "Mechanical Behavior of the Human Lumbar and Lumbosacral Spine as Shown by Three-Dimensional Load-Displacement Curves." *Journal of Bone and Joint Surgery* 76, no. 3 (March 1994): 413–424. https://doi.org/ 10.2106/00004623-199403000-00012.

CHAPTER 10: PATRICIA'S CHRONIC BACK PAIN

How common is back pain? Give a lecture to a crowded room, likely a third of the audience have some right now!

Ma, Vincent Y., Leighton Chan and Kadir J. Carruthers. "Incidence, Prevalence, Costs, and Impact on Disability of Common Conditions Requiring Rehabilitation in the United States." *Archives of Physical Medicine and Rehabilitation* 95, no. 5 (May 2014): 986–995. https://doi.org/10.1016/j.apmr.2013.10.032.

How common is disc degeneration? The majority of adults show some in their imaging.

Teraguchi, M., N. Yoshimura, H. Hashizume, S. Muraki, H. Yamada, A. Minamide, H. Oka, Y. Ishimoto, K. Nagata, R. Kagotani, N. Takiguchi, T. Akune, H. Kawaguchi, K. Nakamura and M. Yoshida. "Prevalence and Distribution of Intervertebral Disc Degeneration Over the Entire Spine in a Population-Based Cohort: The Wakayama Spine Study." *Osteoarthritis and Cartilage* 22, no. 1 (January 2014): 104–110. https://doi.org/10.1016/j.joca.2013.10.019.

What about these epidural spinal injections — are they any good?

Friedly, Janna L., Bryan A. Comstock, Judith A. Turner, Patrick J. Heagerty, Richard A. Deyo, Sean D. Sullivan, Zoya Bauer, Brian W. Bresnahan, Andrew L. Avins, Srdjan S. Nedeljkovic, et al. "A Randomized Trial of Epidural Glucocorticoid Injections for Spinal Stenosis." *New England Journal of Medicine* 371, no. 1 (July 2014): 11–21. https://doi.org/10.1056/NEJMoa1313265.

Narcotics don't work well for chronic pain.

With the current narcotics crisis there's a huge and very active literature on this subject, and here's just a taste of it.

Kalakoti, Piyush, Nathan R. Hendrickson, Nicholas A. Bedard and Andrew J. Pugely. "Opioid Utilization Following Lumbar

Arthrodesis: Trends and Factors Associated with Long-Term Use." *Spine* 43, no. 17 (September 2018): 1208–1216. https://doi.org /10.1097/BRS.0000000000002734.

Raad, Micheal, Amit Jain, Brian J. Neuman, Hamid Hassanzadeh, Munish C. Gupta, Douglas C. Burton, Gregory M. Mundis Jr., Virginie Lafage, Eric O. Klineberg, Richard A. Hostin, Christopher P. Ames, Shay Bess, Daniel M. Sciubba and Khaled M. Kebaish. "Association of Patient-Reported Narcotic Use with Short- and Long-Term Outcomes after Adult Spinal Deformity Surgery: Multicenter Study of 425 Patients with 2-Year Follow-up." *Spine* 43, no. 19 (2018): 1340–1346. https://doi.org /10.1097/BRS.0000000000002631.

How common is lumbar spinal stenosis?

Buser, Zorica, Brandon Ortega, Anthony D'Oro, William Pannell, Jeremiah R. Cohen, Justin Wang, Ray Golish, Michael Reed and Jeffrey C. Wang. "Spine Degenerative Conditions and Their Treatments: National Trends in the United States of America." *Global Spine Journal* 8, no. 1 (February 2018): 57–67. https://doi.org /10.1177/2192568217696688.

Can spinal stenosis — pinched nerves — cause only back pain? And can surgery relieve that?

Mulholland, R.C. "Management of Dural Compressive Syndromes — a Personal History." *The Spine Journal* 17, no. 3 (March 2017): S1–S2. https://doi.org/10.1016/j.spinee.2017.01.005.

CHAPTER 12: ANN THE WIDOW

Most spine pain doesn't need surgery.

Guyer, R.D. and C.W. Hancock. "Chapter 19: Axial Pain and Lumbar Degenerative Disease." In *Orthopedic Knowledge Update: Spine 5*, edited by Eeric Truumees and Heidi Prather, 265–282. Rosemont, Illinois: American Academy of Orthopaedic Surgeons, 2017.

What's the multidisciplinary pain clinic all about?

Big business, big literature. Here's a whole book about this!

Tunks, E. "Chapter 12: Multidisciplinary Pain Clinic Treatment." In *Chronic Pain: A Health Policy Perspective*, edited by Saifudin Rashiq, Donald Schopflocher, Paul Taenzer and Egon Jonsson, 141–152. New York: Wiley-Blackwell, 2018.

Vartiainen, Pekka, Tarja Heiskanen, Harri Sintonen, Risto P. Roine and Eija Kalso. "Health-Related Quality of Life Change in Patients Treated at a Multidisciplinary Pain Clinic." *European Journal of Pain* 23, no. 7 (August 2019): 1318–1328. https://doi.org /10.1002/ejp.1398.

Does a laminectomy create instability — or at least an increased mobility that could lead to instability?

Rao, Raj D., Mei Wang, Peeush Singhal, Linda M. McGrady and Santi Rao. "Intradiscal Pressure and Kinematic Behavior of Lumbar Spine after Bilateral Laminotomy and Laminectomy." *The Spine Journal* 2 (2002): 320–326. https://doi.org/10.1016/s1529-9430(02)00402-3.

What is "spinal balance" and why does it matter?

Glassman, Steven D., Keith Bridwell, John R. Dimar, William Horton, Sigurd Berven and Frank Schwab. "The Impact of Positive Sagittal Balance in Adult Spinal Deformity." *Spine* 38, no. 8 (September 2005): 2024–2029. https://doi.org/10.1097/01.brs .0000179086.30449.96.

Mehta, Vivek A., Anubhav Amin, Ibrahim Omeis, Ziya L. Gokaslan and Oren N. Gottfried. "Implications of Spinopelvic Alignment for the Spine Surgeon." *Neurosurgery* 70, no. 3 (March 2012): 707–721. https://doi.org/10.1227/NEU.0b013e31823262ea.

Diebo, Bassel G., Neil V. Shah, Oheneba Boachie-Adjei, Feng Zhu, Dominique A. Rothenfluh, Carl B. Paulino, Frank J. Schwab and Virginie Lafage. "Adult Spinal Deformity." *Lancet* 394 (July 2019): 160–172. https://doi.org/10.1016/S0140-6736(19)31125-0.

Rothenfluh, Dominique A., Daniel A. Mueller, Esin Rothenfluh and Kan Min. "Pelvic Incidence-Lumbar Lordosis Mismatch Predisposes to Adjacent Segment Disease after Lumbar Spinal Fusion." *European Spine Journal* 24, no. 6 (June 2015): 1251–1258.

Can bone surgeons do anything about the quality of the bones they work on?

Kadri, Aamir, Neil Binkley, Kristyn J. Hare and Paul A. Anderson. "Bone Health Optimization in Orthopedic Surgery." *Journal of Bone and Joint Surgery* 102, no. 7 (April 2020): 574–581. https://doi.org/10.2106/JBJS.19.00999.

What about osteoporosis spine fractures?

Buchbinder, Rachelle, Renea V. Johnston, Kobi J. Rischin, Joanne Homik, C. Allyson Jones, Kamran Golmohammadi and David F. Kallmes. "Percutaneous Vertebroplasty for Osteoporotic Vertebral Compression Fracture." *Cochrane Database Systematic Review* 4, no. 4 (April 2014): CD006349. https://doi.org/10.1002/14651858.

Carragee, Eugene J. "The Vertebroplasty Affair: The Mysterious Case of the Disappearing Effect Size." *The Spine Journal* 10, no. 3 (March 2010): 191–192. https://doi.org/10.1016/j.spinee.2010 .01.002.

Ebeling, Peter R., Kristina Akesson, Douglas C. Bauer, Rachelle Buchbinder, Richard Eastell, Howard A. Fink, Lora Giangregorio, Nuria Guanabens, Deborah Kado, David Kallmes, et al. "The Efficacy and Safety of Vertebral Augmentation: A Second ASBMR Task Force Report." *Journal of Bone and Mineral Research* 34, no. 1 (2019): 3–21. https://doi.org/10.1002/jbmr.3653.

How should a knowledgeable physician examine the low back patient?

"Chapter 8: Examination of the Back." In *Macnab's Backache: Fourth Edition*, edited by David A. Wong and Ensor Transfeldt, 148–165. Philadelphia: Lippincott Williams & Wilkins, 2007.

What is Bertolotti's syndrome?

Tucker, Braden J., Douglas S. Weinberg and Raymond W. Liu. "Lumbosacral Transitional Vertebrae: A Cadaveric Investigation of Prevalence and Relation to Lumbar Degenerative Disease." *Clinical Spine Surgery* 32 (2019): E330–E334. https://doi.org/10.1097/BSD.0000000000000839.

That weird screws-into-the-disc thing I do sometimes.

Bednar, Drew A. and E. Demetra Bednar. "Transosseous Intradiscal Screw Fixation in Lumbar Reconstruction: Clinical Experience with an Alternative in Osteoporosis Fixation." *Clinical Neurology and Neurosurgery* 174 (2018): 187–191. https://doi.org/10.1097/BSD.0000000000000839.

Does managing the osteoporosis make a difference to the lumbar spine fusion patient?

Ohtori, Seiji, Gen Inoue, Sumihisa Orita, Kazuyo Yamauchi, Yawara Eguchi, Nobuyasu Ochiai, Shunji Kishida, Kazuki Kuniyoshi, Yasuchika Aoki, Junichi Nakamura, et al. "Comparison of Teriparatide and Bisphosphonate Treatment to Reduce Pedicle Screw Loosening After Lumbar Spinal Fusion Surgery in Postmenopausal Women with Osteoporosis from a Bone Quality Perspective." *Spine* 38, no. 8 (2013): E487–E492. https://doi.org/10.1097/BRS.0b013e31828826dd.

Ebata, Shigeto, Jun Takahashi, Tomohiko Hasegawa, Keijiro Mukaiyama, Yukihiro Isogai, Tetsuro Ohba, Yosuke Shibata, Toshiyuki Ojima, Zentaro Yamagata, Yukihiro Matsuyama and Hirotaka Haro. "Role of Weekly Teriparatide Administration in

Osseous Union Enhancement within Six Months After Posterior or Transforaminal Lumbar Interbody Fusion for Osteoporosis-Associated Lumbar Degenerative Disorders a Multicenter, Prospective Randomized Study." *Journal of Bone and Joint Surgery* 99, no. 5 (March 2017): 365–372. https://doi.org/10.2106/JBJS.16.00230.

CHAPTER 13: MELINDA THE ACTIVE RETIREE

What is discitis and how are these spine infections best treated?

Boody, Barrett S., Tyler J. Jenkins, Joseph Maslak, Wellington K. Hsu and Alpesh A. Patel. "Vertebral Osteomyelitis and Spinal Epidural Abscess: An Evidence-Based Review." *Journal of Spinal Disorders and Technique* 28, no. 6 (July 2015): E316–E327. https://doi.org/10.1097/BSD.0000000000000294.

On spinal instability.

Panjabi, M.M., T.R. Oxland, I. Yamamoto and J.J. Crisco. "Mechanical Behavior of the Human Lumbar and Lumbosacral Spine as Shown by Three-Dimensional Load-Displacement Curves." *Journal of Bone and Joint Surgery* 76 (March 1994): 413–424.

Successful implant treatment of spine infections.

Ruf, Michael, Dieter Stoltze, Harry R. Merk, Michael Ames and Jürgen Harms. "Treatment of Vertebral Osteomyelitis by Radical Debridement and Stabilization Using Titanium Mesh Cages." *Spine* 32, no. 9 (April 2007): E275–E280. https://doi.org/10.1097/01.brs.0000261034.83395.7f.

Hey, Hwee Weng Dennis, Li Wen Nathaniel Ng, Chuen Seng Tan, Dale Fisher, Anupama Vasudevan, Ka-Po Gabriel Liu, Joseph Shantakumar Thambiah, Naresh Kumar, Leok-Lim Lau, Hee-Kit Wong and Paul Anantharajah Tambyah. "Spinal Implants Can Be

Inserted in Patients with Deep Spine Infection." *Spine* 42, no. 8 (April 2017): E490–E495. https://doi.org/10.1097/BRS .0000000000001747.

CHAPTER 14: MAX THE MECHANIC

How well can you recover from a badly symptomatic spinal cord compression?

OK, these articles all go to the neck where this problem is most common. Max's case in the T-spine was relatively rare and most of the literature there goes to disc hernia, which was not Max's problem. Spinal cord is spinal cord and really they behave the same in the clinic, and afterwards.

Nurick, S. "The Natural History and the Results of Surgical Treatment of the Spinal Cord Disorder Associated with Cervical Spondylosis." *Brain* 95, no. 1 (January 1972): 101–108. https://doi.org /10.1093/brain/95.1.101.

Kopjar, Branko, Parker E. Bohm, Joshua H. Arnold, Michael G. Fehlings, Lindsay A. Tetreault and Paul M. Arnold. "Outcomes of Surgical Decompression in Patients with Very Severe Degenerative Cervical Myelopathy." *Spine* 43, no. 16 (August 2018): 1102–1109. https://doi.org/10.1097/BRS.0000000000002602.

Tetreault, Lindsay A., Pierre Côté, Branko Kopjar, Paul Arnold and Michael G. Fehlings. "A Clinical Prediction Model to Assess Surgical Outcome in Patients with Cervical Spondylotic Myelopathy: Internal and External Validations Using the Prospective Multicenter Aospine North American and International Datasets of 743 Patients." *The Spine Journal* 15 (March 2015): 388–397. https://doi.org/10.1016/j.spinee.2014.12.145.

What determines how well the half-paralyzed patient will recover?

Nakashima, Hiroaki, Yasutsugu Yukawa, Keigo Ito, Masaaki Machino, Shunsuke Kanbara, Daigo Morita, Hiroshi Takahashi,

Shiro Imagama, Zenya Ito, Naoki Ishiguro and Fumihiko Kato. "Prediction of Lower Limb Functional Recovery after Laminoplasty for Cervical Myelopathy: Focusing on the 10-S Step Test." *European Spine Journal* 21, no. 7 (March 2012): 1389–1395. https://doi.org/10.1007/s00586-012-2241-z.

Karadimas, Spyridon K., W. Mark Erwin, Claire G. Ely, Joseph R. Dettori and Michael G. Fehlings. "Pathophysiology and Natural History of Cervical Spondylotic Myelopathy." *Spine* 38 (October 2013): S21–S36. https://doi.org/10.1097/BRS.0b013e3182a7f2c3.

Yoon, S. Tim, Annie Raich, Robin E. Hashimoto, K. Daniel Riew, Christopher I. Shaffrey, John M. Rhee, Lindsay A. Tetreault, Andrea C. Skelly and Michael G. Fehlings. "Predictive Factors Affecting Outcome after Cervical Laminoplasty." *Spine* 38, no. S1 (October 2013): S232–S252. https://doi.org/10.1097/BRS.0b013e3182a7eb55.

CHAPTER 15: NORONHA THE NURSE

How common is bad degeneration in the neck without symptoms?

Bednarik, Josef, Zdenek Kadanka, Ladislav Dusek, Oldrich Novotny, Dagmar Surelova, Igor Urbanek and Boleslav Prokes. "Presymptomatic Spondylotic Cervical Cord Compression." *Spine* 29. No. 20 (October 2004): 2260–2269. https://doi.org/10.1097/01.brs.0000142434.02579.84.

What is the Gore angle in cervical collapse?

Katsuura, Yoshihiro, Alex Lemons, Eileen Lorenz, Rachel Swafford, James Osborn and Garrick Cason. "Radiographic Analysis of Cervical and Spinal Alignment in Multilevel ACDF with Lordotic Interbody Device." *International Journal of Spine Surgery* 11, no. 2 (April 2017): 91–98. https://doi.org/10.14444/4013.

Chavanne, Albert, David B. Pettigrew, Jeffrey R. Holtz, Neal Dollin and Charles Kuntz. "Spinal Cord Intramedullary Pressure in Cervical Kyphotic Deformity: A Cadaveric Study." *Spine* 36, no. 20 (2011): 1619–1626.

Gore, Donald, Susan B. Sepic and Gena Gardner. "Roentgenographic Findings of the Cervical Spine in Asymptomatic People." *Spine* 11, no. 6 (1986): 521–524. https://doi.org/10.1097/00007632 -198607000-00003.

What is cervical deformity?

Cho, Samuel K., Scott Safir, Joseph M. Lombardi and Jun S. Kim. "Cervical Spine Deformity: Indications, Consideration and Surgical Outcomes." *Journal of the American Academy of Orthopedic Surgery* 27, no. 12 (June 2019): e555–e567. https://doi.org/0.5435 /JAAOS-D-17-00546.

How common is CSM?

Nouri, Aria, Lindsay Tetreault, Anoushka Singh, Spyridon K. Karadimas and Michael G. Fehlings. "Degenerative Cervical Myelopathy: Epidemiology, Genetics and Pathogenesis." *Spine* 40, no. 12 (June 2015): E675–E693. https://doi.org/10.1097/BRS .0000000000000913.

Fehlings, Michael G., Lindsay A. Tetreault, Jefferson R. Wilson and Andrea C. Skelly. "Cervical Spondylotic Myelopathy: Current State of the Art and Future Directions." *Spine* 38, no. 22S (October 2013): S1–S8. https://doi.org/10.1097/BRS.0b013e3182a7e9e0.

Is surgery any better done from the front versus posterior approach?

Cunningham, Mary R.A., Stuart Hershman and John Bendo. "Systematic Review of Cohort Studies Comparing Surgical Treatments for Cervical Spondylotic Myelopathy." *Spine* 35, no. 5 (March 2010): 537–543. https://doi.org/10.1097/BRS .0b013e3181b204cc.

Lawrence, Brandon D., W. Bradley Jacobs, Daniel C. Norvell, Jeffrey
T. Hermsmeyer, Jens R. Chapman and Darrel S. Brodke. "Anterior
Versus Posterior Approach for Treatment of Cervical Spondylotic
Myelopathy: A Systematic Review." *Spine* 38, no. 22S (October 2013):
S173–S182. https://doi.org/10.1097/BRS.0b013e3182a7eaaf.

Fehlings, Michael G., Sean Barry, Branko Kopjar, Sangwook Tim
Yoon, Paul Arnold, Eric M. Massicotte, Alexander Vaccaro, Darrel
S. Brodke, Christopher Shaffrey, Justin S. Smith, Eric Woodard,
Robert J. Banco, Jens Chapman, Michael Janssen, Christopher
Bono, Rick Sasso, Mark Dekutoski and Ziya L Gokaslan.
"Anterior Versus Posterior Surgical Approaches to Treat Cervical
Spondylotic Myelopathy: Outcomes of the Prospective Multicenter
AO Spine North America CSM Study in 264 Patients." *Spine* 28,
no. 26 (December 2013): 2247–2252. https://doi.org/10.1097/BRS
.0000000000000047.

CHAPTER 16: SARAH'S STORY

What's the best imaging for a suspected spine cancer?

Shah, Lubdha M. and Karen L. Salzman. "Imaging of Spinal Metastatic
Disease." *International Journal of Surgical Oncology* 1 (2011): 1–12.

How well does surgery work in metastatic spine cancer even when you're halfway paralyzed?

Patchell, Roy A., Phillip A. Tibbs, William F. Regine, Richard Payne,
Stephen Saris, Richard J. Kryscio, Mohammed Mohiuddin and
Byron Young. "Direct Decompressive Surgical Resection in the
Treatment of Spinal Cord Compression Caused by Metastatic
Cancer: A Randomised Trial." *Lancet* 366 (2005): 643–648. https://
doi.org/10.1016/S0140-6736(05)66954-1.

Lee, Chang-Hyun, Ji-Woong Kwon, Jaebong Lee, Seung-Jae Hyun,
Ki-Jeong Kim, Tae-Ahn Jahng and Hyun-Jib Kim. "Direct

Decompressive Surgery Followed by Radiotherapy Versus Radiotherapy Alone for Metastatic Epidural Spinal Cord Compression: A Meta-analysis." *Spine* 39, no. 9 (April 2014): E587–E592. https://doi.org/10.1097/BRS.0000000000000258.

CHAPTER 17: MORRIS'S LOW BACK MIRACLE

How common is an asymptomatic disc bulge? Roughly equal to your age in years!

Boden, S.D., P.R. McCowin, D.O. Davis, T.S. Dina, A.S. Mark and S.W. Wiesel. "Abnormal Magnetic Resonance Scans of the Lumbar Spine in Asymptomatic Subjects." *Journal of Bone and Joint Surgery* 72, no. 3 (March 1990): 403–408.

Does every disc hernia need surgery — what happens without? What is the "natural history"?

Wong, J.J., P. Côté, D.A. Sutton, K. Randhawa, H. Yu, S. Varatharajan, R. Goldgrub, M. Nordin, D.P. Gross, H.M. Shearer, L.J. Carroll, P.J. Stern, A. Ameis, D. Southerst, S. Mior, M. Stupar, T. Varatharajan and A. Taylor-Vaisey. "Clinical Practice Guidelines for the Noninvasive Management of Low Back Pain: A Systematic Review by the Ontario Protocol for Traffic Injury Management. (OPTIMa) Collaboration." *European Journal of Pain* 21, no. 2 (2017): 201–216. https://doi.org/10.1002/ejp.931.

Dagenais, Simon, Andrea C. Tricco and Scott Haldeman. "Synthesis of Recommendations for the Assessment and Management of Low Back Pain from Recent Clinical Practice Guidelines." *The Spine Journal* 10, no. 6 (2010): 514–529. https://doi.org/10.1016/j.spinee.2010.03.032.

Epidural steroids for disc hernia.

Osterman, Heikki, Seppo Seitsalo, Jaro Karppinen and Antti Malmivaara. "Effectiveness of Microdiscectomy for Lumbar Disc

Herniation: A Randomized Controlled Trial with 2 Years of
Follow-Up." *Spine* 31, no. 21 (October 2006): 2409–2414. https://
doi.org/10.1097/01.brs.0000239178.08796.52.

Buttermann, Glen R. "Treatment of Lumbar Disc Herniation:
Epidural Steroid Injection Compared with Discectomy: A
Prospective, Randomized Study." *Journal of Bone and Joint Surgery*
86, no. 4 (April 2004): 670–679.

What is this minimally invasive surgery (MIS) thing?

Rasouli, Mohammad R., Vafa Rahimi-Movaghar, Farhad Shokraneh,
Maziar Moradi-Lakeh and Roger Chou. "Minimally Invasive
Discectomy Versus Microdiscectomy/Open Discectomy for
Symptomatic Lumbar Disc Herniation." *Cochrane Database
Systematic Reviews* 4, no. 9 (September 2014): CD010328. https://
doi.org/10.1002/14651858.CD010328.pub2.

Is MIS any better than open surgery?

"Minimally Invasive Hype?" *The Back Letter* 34, no. 10 (October 2019):
109–118. https://doi.org/10.1097/01.BACK.0000585348.09540.08.

Anderson, P.A. "Evidence-Based Orthopedics: Tubular Discectomy
Resulted in Greater Leg and Back Pain and a Lower Rate of
Recovery Than Conventional Microdiscectomy for Sciatica."
Journal of Bone and Joint Surgery 92 (2010): 475.

Evaniew, Nathan, Moin Khan, Brian Drew, Desmond Kwok, Mohit
Bhandari and Michelle Ghert. "Minimally Invasive Versus Open
Surgery for Cervical and Lumbar Discectomy: A Systematic
Review and Meta-analysis." *Canadian Medical Association Journal
Open* 2, no. 4 (October 2014): E295–E305. https://doi.org/10.9778
/cmajo.20140048.

Should we worry that something else is going on when disc surgery doesn't go right?

Boutin, Pierre and Howard Hogshead. "Surgical Pathology of the Intervertebral Disc: Is Routine Examination Necessary?" *Spine* 17, no. 10 (October 1992): 1236–1238. https://doi.org/10.1097/00007632 -199210000-00018.

Grzybicki, Dana M., Edward J. Callaghan and Stephen S. Raab. "Cost-Benefit Value of Microscopic Examination of Intervertebral Discs." *Journal of Neurosurgery* 89 (1998): 378–381. https://doi.org/10.3171/jns.1998.89.3.0378.

Reddy, Praveen, Ray Williams, Brian Willis and Anil Nanda. "Pathological Evaluation of Intervertebral Disc Tissue Specimens after Routine Cervical and Lumbar Decompression: A Cost-Benefit Analysis Retrospective Study." *Surgical Neurology* 56 (2001): 252–255. https://doi.org/10.1016/S0090-3019(01)00585-7.

Wu, Adam S. and Daryl R. Fourney. "Histopathological Examination of Intervertebral Disc Specimens: A Cost-Benefit Analysis." *Canadian Journal of Neurological Science* 34 (2007): 451–455. https://doi.org/10.1017/s0317167100007344.

CHAPTER 18: MARIA'S STORY

Why does flexion of the body relieve symptoms in spinal stenosis?

Fujiwara, Atsushi, Howard S. An, Tae-Hong Lim and Victor M. Haughton. "Morphologic Changes in the Lumbar Intervertebral Foramen Due to Fexion-Extension, Lateral Bending, and Axial Rotation: An In Vitro Anatomic and Biomechanical Study." *Spine* 26, no. 8 (April 2001): 876–882. https://doi.org/10.1097/00007632 -200104150-00010.

Spivak, Jeffrey M., Frederick J. Kummer, Deyu Chen, Martin Quirno and Jonathan R. Kamerlink. "Intervertebral Foramen Size and Volume Changes in Low Grade, Low Dysplasia Isthmic Spondylolisthesis." *Spine* 35, no. 20 (September 2010): 1829–1835. https://doi.org/10.1097/BRS.0b013e3181ccc59d.

Is there really a deficit in musculoskeletal medical education? Spine is musculoskeletal!

Goff, Ian, Elspeth Mary Wise, David Coady and David Walker. "Musculoskeletal Training: Are GP Trainees Exposed to the Right Case Mix for Independent Practice?" *Clinical Rheumatology* 35, no. 2 (February 2016): 507–511. https://doi.org/10.1007/s10067-014-2767-z.

Murphy, Robert F., Dawn M. LaPorte and Veronica M.R. Wadey. "Current Concepts Review. Musculoskeletal Education in Medical School: Deficits in Knowledge and Strategies for Improvement." *Journal of Bone and Joint Surgery* 96, no. 23 (December 2014): 2009–2014. https://doi.org/10.2106/JBJS.N.00354.

Those two first seminal articles from 1911 on back pain/fusion surgery.

These are reproduced in a 2007 Focus edition of the journal *Clinical Orthopedics and Related Research*, which I have referenced here. All the articles in this symposium are free downloads from the journal website.

Albee, Fred H. "Transplantation of a Portion of the Tibia into the Spine for Pott's Disease: A Preliminary Report (1911)." *Clinical Orthopedics and Related Research* 460 (July 2007): 14–16. https://doi.org/10.1097/BLO.0b013e3180686a0f.

Hibbs, Russell A. "An Operation for Progressive Spinal Deformities: A Preliminary Report of Three Cases from the Service of the Orthopaedic Hospital (1911)." *Clinical Orthopedics and Related Research* 460 (July 2007): 17–20. https://doi.org/10.1097/BLO.0b013e3180686b30.

Early key research on lateral recess stenosis.

Postacchini, F., G. Cinotti, D. Perugia and S. Gumina. "The Surgical Treatment of Central Lumbar Stenosis. Multiple Laminotomy

Compared with Total Laminectomy." *Journal of Bone and Joint Surgery* 75, no. 3 (May 1993): 386–392. https://doi.org/10.1302/0301 -620X.75B3.8496205.

Postacchini, F. "Surgical Management of Lumbar Spinal Stenosis." *Spine* 24, no. 10 (May 1999): 1043–1047. https://doi.org/10.1097 /00007632-199905150-00020.

CHAPTER 19: JACK'S BACK-BREAKING JOB

Workers' compensation back pain surgery doesn't do so well.

"Increasingly Honest Portrayals of the Role of Fusion for Back Pain and Disc Degeneration." *The Back Letter* 32, no. 7 (July 2017): 76–77. https://doi.org/10.1097/01.BACK.0000520974.25033.23.

Epidural injections aren't great for chronic back pain either.

Young, Lu, Javier Z. Guzman, Devina Purmessur, James C. Iatridis, Andrew C. Hecht, Sheeraz A. Qureshi and Samuel K. Cho. "Nonoperative Management of Discogenic Back Pain: A Systematic Review." *Spine* 39, no. 16 (2014): 1314–1324. https://doi .org/10.1097/BRS.0000000000000401.

Successful outcomes of fusion for "nonspecific" low back pain from disc degeneration without instability, neurological compression of malalignment run around 70 percent.

Kleimeyer, John P., Ivan Cheng, Todd F. Alamin, Serena S. Hu, Thomas Cha, Vijay Yanamadala and Kirkham B. Wood. "Selective Anterior Lumbar Interbody Fusion for Low Back Pain Associated with Degenerative Disc Disease Versus Nonsurgical Management." *Spine* 43, no. 19 (October 2018): 1372–1380. https://doi.org/10.1097/BRS.0000000000002630.

Internal lumbar disc derangement (ILDD) is a better indicator for fusion surgery.

Lee, Casey K., Paul Vessa and June Kyu Lee. "Chronic Disabling Low Back Pain Syndrome Caused by Internal Disc Derangements: The Results of Disc Excision and Posterior Lumbar Interbody Fusion." *Spine* 20, no. 3 (February 1995): 356–360. https://doi.org/10.1097/00007632-199502000-00018.

What are these "Modic" changes?

Modic, M.T., P.M. Steinberg, J.S. Ross, T.J. Masaryk and J.R. Carter. "Degenerative Disc Disease: Assessment of Changes in Vertebral Bone Marrow with MR Imaging." *Radiology* 166 (January 1988): 193–199. https://doi.org/10.1148/radiology.166.1.3336678.

Is the (very macro-invasive, but I don't care because we should all be much more interested in maximally effective than in minimally invasive) PLIF operation a good thing?

Suk, Se-II, Choon-Ki Lee, Won-Joong Kim, Ji-Ho Lee, Kyu-Jung Cho and Hyung-Gook Kim. "Adding Posterior Lumbar Interbody Fusion to Pedicle Screw Fixation and Posterolateral Fusion After Decompression in Spondylolytic Spondylolisthesis." *Spine* 22, no. 2 (January 1997): 210–220. https://doi.org/10.1097/00007632-199701150-00016.

What is the impact of alignment on fusion outcomes?

Glassman, Steven D., Keith Bridwell, John R. Dimar, William Horton, Sigurd Berven and Frank Schwab. "The Impact of Positive Sagittal Balance in Adult Spinal Deformity." *Spine* 38, no. 8 (September 2005): 2024–2029. https://doi.org/10.1097/01.brs.0000179086.30449.96.

Cardiac risk is a thing in major spine surgery.

Faciszewski, Ton, Ron Jensen, Roxann Rokey and Richard Berg. "Cardiac Risk Stratification of Patients with Symptomatic Spinal

Stenosis." *Clinical Orthopedics and Related Research* 384 (March 2001): 110–115. https://doi.org/10.1097/00003086-200103000-00013

Carabini, Louanne M., Carine Zeeni, Natalie C. Moreland, Robert W. Gould, Laura B. Hemmer, John F. Bebawy, Tyler R. Koski, Jamal McClendon Jr., Antoun Koht and Dhanesh K. Gupta. "Predicting Major Adverse Cardiac Events in Spine Fusion Patients: Is the Revised Cardiac Risk Index Sufficient?" *Spine* 39, no. 17 (August 2014): 1441–1448. https://doi.org/10.1097/BRS .0000000000000405.

Your doctor likely didn't learn much about your back in medical school.

Murphy, Robert F., Dawn M. LaPorte and Veronica M.R. Wadey. "Current Concepts Review. Musculoskeletal Education in Medical School: Deficits in Knowledge and Strategies for Improvement." *Journal of Bone and Joint Surgery* 96, no. 23 (December 2014): 2009–2014. https://doi.org/10.2106/JBJS.N.00354.

CHAPTER 20: THEO DIDN'T GET BETTER

Does surgery at the wrong level really happen?

Mody, Milan G., Ali Nourbakhsh, Daniel L. Stahl, Mark Gibbs, Mohammad Alfawareh and Kim J. Garges. "The Prevalence of Wrong Level Surgery among Spine Surgeons." *Spine* 33, no. 2 (January 2008): 194–198. https://doi.org/10.1097/BRS.0b013e31816043d1.

Irace, Claudio and Susanna Usai. "The 'Nightmare' of Wrong Level in Spine Surgery: A Critical Appraisal." *Patient Safety in Surgery* 6 (June 2012): 14.

What is the expected benefit of spinal cord decompression surgery?

Fehlings, Michael G., Lindsay A. Tetreault, Jefferson R. Wilson and Andrea C. Skelly. "Cervical Spondylotic Myelopathy: Current

State of the Art and Future Directions." *Spine* 38, no. 22S
(October 2013): S1–S8. https://doi.org/10.1097/BRS
.0b013e3182a7e9e0.

The role of parallel bars in spinal cord rehab.

Visintin, M. and H. Barbeau. "The Effects of Parallel Bars, Body
Weight Support and Speed on the Modulation of the Locomotor
Pattern of Spastic Paretic Gait: A Preliminary Communication."
Spinal Cord 32 (1994): 540–553. https://doi.org/10.1038/sc.1994.86.

CHAPTER 21: RICARDO'S WRECKAGE

Anatomy of spinal stenosis — central versus lateral.

Lee, Casey K., Wolfgang Rauschning and William Glenn. "Lateral
Lumbar Spinal Canal Stenosis: Classification, Pathologic
Anatomy and Surgical Decompression." *Spine* 13, no. 3 (1988):
313–320.

Van Akkerveeken, Pieter F. "Classification of Canal and Lateral
Stenosis of the Lumbar Spine." In *Lumbar Spinal Stenosis*, edited
by R. Gunzberg and M. Szpalski, 49–60. Philadelphia: Lippincott
Williams & Wilkins, 2000.

Crock, H.V. "Normal and Pathological Anatomy of the Lumbar
Spinal Nerve Root Canals." *Journal of Bone and Joint Surgery* 13,
no. 4 (1981): 79–83. https://doi.org/10.1302/0301-620X.63B4.7298672.

Why bending forward opens your nerve tunnels.

Fujiwara, Atsushi, Howard S. An, Tae-Hong Lim and Victor M.
Haughton. "Morphologic Changes in the Lumbar Intervertebral
Foramen Due to Fexion-Extension, Lateral Bending, and Axial
Rotation: An In Vitro Anatomic and Biomechanical Study." *Spine*
26, no. 8 (April 2001): 876–882. https://doi.org/10.1097/00007632
-200104150-00010.

The odds of the surgical spine care patient coming back for more.

Hilibrand, Alan S., Gregory Carlson, Mark A. Palumbo and Paul K. Jones. "Radiculopathy and Myelopathy at Segments Adjacent to the Site of a Previous Anterior Cervical Arthrodesis." *Journal of Bone and Joint Surgery* 81, no. 4 (1999): 519–528.

What is postlaminectomy instability?

Mosenthal, William P., Jason L. Dickherber, Bradley H. Saitta and Michael J. Lee. "Post Laminectomy Instability." *Seminars in Spine Surgery* 31, no. 3 (April 2019): 100173. https://doi.org/10.1053/j.semss.2019.04.007.

All about optimal spinal alignment.

Mehta, Vivek A., Anubhav Amin, Ibrahim Omeis, Ziya L. Gokaslan and Oren N. Gottfried. "Implications of Spinopelvic Alignment for the Spine Surgeon." *Neurosurgery* 70, no. 3 (March 2012): 707–721. https://doi.org/10.1227/NEU.0b013e31823262ea.

Diebo, Bassel G., Neil V. Shah, Oheneba Boachie-Adjei, Feng Zhu, Dominique A. Rothenfluh, Carl B. Paulino, Frank J. Schwab and Virginie Lafage. "Adult Spinal Deformity." *Lancet* 394 (July 2019): 160–172. https://doi.org/10.1016/S0140-6736(19)31125-0.

Four rods may be better than two.

Shen, Francis H., Daniel Woods, Matthew Miller, Brian Murrell and Sasi Vadapalli. "Use of the Dual Construct Lowers Rod Strains in Flexion-Extension and Lateral Bending Compared to Two-Rod and Two-Rod Satellite Constructs in a Cadaveric Spine Corpectomy Model." *The Spine Journal* 12 (2021): 2104–2111. https://doi.org/10.1016/j.spinee.2021.05.022.

Vosoughi, Ardalan Seyed, Amin Joukar, Ali Kiapour, Dikshya Parajuli, Anand K. Agarwal, Vijay K. Goel and Joseph Zavatsky. "Optimal Satellite Rod Constructs to Mitigate Rod Failure

Following Pedicle Subtraction Osteotomy (POS): A Finite Element Study." *The Spine Journal* 19, no. 5 (2018): 931–941. https://doi.org/10.1016/j.spinee.2018.11.003.

How loads on the spine vary with posture.

Nachemsen, A., and J.M. Morris. "In Vivo Measurements of Intradiscal Pressure." *Journal of Bone and Joint Surgery* 46 (1964): 1077–1092.

Alexander, Lyndsay A., Elizabeth Hancock, Ioannis Agouris, Francis W. Smith and Alasdair MacSween. "The Response of the Nucleus Pulposus of the Lumbar Intervertebral Discs to Functionally Loaded Positions." *Spine* 32, no. 14 (June 2007): 1508–1512. https://doi.org/10.1097/BRS.0b013e318067dccb.

A third of people with spinal stenosis have unstable spines even before their surgery!

Segebarth, Brad, Mark F. Kurd, Priscilla H. Haug and Rick Davis. "Routine Upright Imaging for Evaluating Degenerative Lumbar Stenosis Incidence of Degenerative Spondylolisthesis Missed on Supine MRI." *Journal of Spinal Disorders and Techniques* 28 (December 2015): 394–397. https://doi.org/10.1097/BSD .0000000000000205.

The North American Spine Society low back X-ray recommendations.

North American Spine Society. "Evidence-Based Clinical Guidelines for Multidisciplinary Spine Care: Diagnosis and Treatment of Degenerative Lumbar Spondylolisthesis." Revised 2014. https://www.spine.org/Portals/O/Documents/ResearchClinicalCare /Guidelines/Spondylolisthesis.pdf.

Cervical spondylotic myelopathy incidence 605/M/yr.

Nouri, Aria, Lindsay Tetreault, Anoushka Singh, Spyridon K. Karadimas and Michael G. Fehlings. "Degenerative Cervical

Myelopathy: Epidemiology, Genetics and Pathogenesis." *Spine* 40, no. 12 (June 2015): E675–E693. https://doi.org/10.1097/BRS .0000000000000913.

Guillain-Barré incidence 0.4-1.7/M/yr.

Alter, Milton. "The Epidemiology of Guillain-Barré Syndrome." *Annals of Neurology* 27, no. S1 (1990): S7–S12. https://doi.org/10.1002/ana .410270704.

Why we should think more about laminectomy than we do . . .

Rao, Raj D., Mei Wang, Peeush Singhal, Linda M. McGrady and Santi Rao. "Intradiscal Pressure and Kinematic Behavior of Lumbar Spine after Bilateral Laminotomy and Laminectomy." *The Spine Journal* 2 (2002): 320–326. https://doi.org/10.1016/s1529 -9430(02)00402-3.

Penicillin allergies most often aren't.

Sarfani, Shumaila, Cosby A. Stone Jr., G. Andrew Murphy and David R. Richardson. "Understanding Penicillin Allergy, Cross-reactivity, and Antibiotic Selection in the Preoperative Setting." *Journal of the American Academy of Orthopedic Surgery* 30, no. 1 (January 2022): e1–e5. https://doi.org/10.5435/JAAOS-D-21-00422.

REFERENCES TO SUPPORT PART 3: SPINE CARE SOLUTIONS

Lynch, T. Sean, Justin E. Hellwinkel, Charles M. Jobin and William N. Levine. "Curriculum Reform and New Technology to Fill the Void of Musculoskeletal Education in the Medical School Curriculum." *Journal of the American Academy of Orthopedic Surgeons* 28 (Decmber 2020): 945–952. https://doi.org/10.5435 /JAAOS-D-20-00485.

Murphy, Robert F., Dawn M. LaPorte and Veronica M.R. Wadey. "Current Concepts Review. Musculoskeletal Education in Medical

School: Deficits in Knowledge and Strategies for Improvement."
Journal of Bone and Joint Surgery 96, no. 23 (December 2014):
2009–2014. https://doi.org/10.2106/JBJS.N.00354.

Aebi, Max. "Education Program of EuroSpine/The Spine Society of
Europe." *European Spine Journal* 19 (December 2010): 1–2.

Gladwell, Malcolm. *Outliers.* Boston: Little, Brown and Company, 2008.

Index

back pain and back-dominant pain —
    surgery
    error in, 187–89, 190
    non-recovery from, 184–87, 190
    skepticism of, 37, 84, 166, 170, 173,
        176, 204
    as solution, 94, 105–6, 165, 168–69,
        170, 204–5
Barr, Dr., xviii
Bednar, Drew
    background and as spine surgeon,
        xiii–xvi
    back problem of, 228–29
    education as spine surgeon, vii
    first encounter with modern
        spine care, vii–xi
    lectures on spine care, 215, 216
    mentors and influences, 239–44
biology, understanding of, 228
biomechanics of patients, 208
bladder, 21, 26, 57, 58, 125
blood counts, 68
bone marrow, 84, 177
bones, 112, 117
bone spur(s)
    development, 11, 12, 128
    in neck, 14
    non-recovery from surgery, 184–87,
        190
    pinching by, 53, 76, 182, 187
    trimming of, xix, 53, 77, 172,
        183–85
bone surgery of spine, history, xvii–xix
bony posterior facet joints infections
    (facet pyarthrosis), 117
BPH (benign prostatic hyperplasia),
    125
brace, 112–13, 201
BritSpine (UK), 219
burning pain, as red flag, 222
burst fracture, as injury, vii–viii
buttocks, and pain, 40, 50, 98

cages, as support devices, 197
Canadian healthcare systems,
    problems in, xi, 15–16
canal (spinal canal)
    impact of tumor, 57
    and laminectomy, 64, 67
    problems in, 11–12
    swollen facet joints in, 193
cancer
    case studies, 55–60, 142–48
    metastatic spine care, 58–60, 98
    and neck problems, 143–44
    and pain, 98
    removal, 142, 146
    in spine, 98, 143, 145
    in thoracic spine, 57–59, 144–47,
        207
cardiology issues for surgery, 77,
    79–80
carpal tunnel, description and role,
    9–10
carpal tunnel syndrome (CTS)
    description, 9, 10
    as diagnosis, 5, 8, 10, 62–63
    misdiagnosis, 70
    splint for, 10
cars, and spine, 233
case studies
    back pain and back-dominant
        pain, 18–27, 28–37, 90–96,
        106–14, 124–30
    cancer, 55–60, 142–48
    compensation clients, 173–80
    crooked artery in neck, 131–41
    infections (spinal), 115–23
    minimally invasive surgical
        technology (MIS), 149–59
    myelopathy, 3–17
    nerve pain, 72–80
    sciatica, 38–46
    spinal alignment, 191–202
    spinal cord surgery, 61–71

This book is also available as a Global Certified Accessible™ (GCA) ebook. ECW Press's ebooks are screen reader friendly and are built to meet the needs of those who are unable to read standard print due to blindness, low vision, dyslexia, or a physical disability.

At ECW Press, we want you to enjoy our books in whatever format you like. If you've bought a print copy, just send an email to ebook@ecwpress .com and include:

- the book title
- the name of the store where you purchased it
- a screenshot or picture of your order/receipt number and your name
- your preference of file type: PDF (for desktop reading), ePub (for a phone/tablet, Kobo, or Nook), mobi (for Kindle)

A real person will respond to your email with your ebook attached. Please note this offer is only for copies bought for personal use and does not apply to school or library copies.

Thank you for supporting an independently owned Canadian publisher with your purchase!

This book is made of paper from well-managed FSC® - certified forests, recycled materials, and other controlled sources.

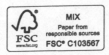
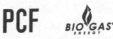